LaFleur Brooks'

Health Unit
COORDINATING

POCKET GUIDE

Second Edition

D0112251

LaFleur Brooks'

Health Unit
COORDINATING
POCKET GUIDE

Elaine A. Gillingham, AAS, BA, CHUC
Program Director 1993–2005 (retired)
Health Unit Coordinator Program
GateWay Community College
Phoenix, Arizona

Monica Wadsworth Seibel, BS, MEd, CHUC
Program Director
Health Unit Coordinator Program
GateWay Community College
Phoenix, Arizona

Second Edition

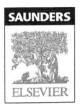

SAUNDERS

ELSEVIER

SAUNDERS
ELSEVIER

The Curtis Center
170 South Independence Mall West, 300E
Philadelphia, Pennsylvania 19106-3399

LaFleur Brooks' Health Unit Coordinating Pocket Guide   ISBN-13: 978-1-4160-5211-1
Copyright © 2009 by W.B. Saunders Company

Notice

Medicine is an ever-changing field. Standard safety precautions must be followed, but as new research and clinical experience broaden our knowledge, changes in treatment and drug therapy may become necessary or appropriate. Readers are advised to check the most current product information provided by the manufacturer of each drug to be administered to verify the recommended dose, the method and duration of administration, and contraindications. It is the responsibility of the treating physician, relying on experience and knowledge of the patient, to determine dosages and the best treatment for each individual patient. Neither the Publisher nor the editor assume any liability for any injury and/or damage to persons or property arising from this publication.

Previous edition copyrighted 2004

ISBN-13: 978-1-4160-5211-1

Publishing Director: Andrew Allen
Acquisitions Editor: Jennifer Allen
Senior Developmental Editor: Ellen Wurm-Cutter
Publishing Services Manager: Julie Eddy
Project Manager: Andrea Campbell
Designer: Julia Dummitt

Working together to grow
libraries in developing countries
www.elsevier.com | www.bookaid.org | www.sabre.org

ELSEVIER   BOOK AID International   Sabre Foundation

Transferred to Digital Printing 2018

Last digit is the print number: 9 8 7 6 5 4 3

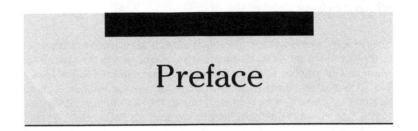

Preface

The *LaFleur Brooks' Health Unit Coordinating Pocket Guide*, Second Edition, is designed to provide assistance to both new and working health unit coordinators. It may be used as a quick reference as well as a personal planner and notebook.

There are many differerent computer ordering systems, forms, and methods of performing tasks among hospitals and units within hospitals nationwide. Many hospitals have implemented the electronic medical record with computer physician order entry, which has expanded the HUC position in other areas. Blank pages have been included to make important notes specific to your hospital/unit for future reference. The history of health unit coordinating and information regarding the National Association of Health Unit Coordinators is included. Health unit coordinator certification and recertification information is also included. Other information vital to the health unit coordinator includes:

- Interpersonal communication
- Use of communication devices
- Maintenance of the patient's paper and electronic chart
- Workplace behavior
- Ethics
- Legal issues—Health Insurance Portability and Accountability Act (HIPAA) laws
- Infection control, emergencies, incident reports
- Transcription of doctors' orders
- Computer physician order entry
- Electronic medical records
- Admission, discharge, and transfer procedures
- Reference lists including a glossary of terms used in the hospital setting, abbreviations, medical terminology word parts, medical/surgical/diagnostic terms, common laboratory procedures, and common medications
- Record-keeping forms are provided for:
    Frequently called telephone numbers
    Clinical notes
    Weekly planner
    Monthly planner

The *LaFleur Brooks' Health Unit Coordinating Pocket Guide* is not intended to replace the health unit coordinating textbooks used in the classroom. Important information has been summarized from *LaFleur Brooks' Health Unit Coordinating*, Sixth Edition, to serve as a quick reference; more detailed information may be researched in the sixth edition. Both new and seasoned health unit coordinators will find this *Pocket Guide* to be a valuable and convenient tool.

Elaine Gillingham
Monica Wadsworth Seibel

Contents

CHAPTER 1

Understanding Health Unit Coordinating

The Health Unit Coordinator Profession

The health unit coordinator (HUC), who is usually the first person seen when one is walking onto a hospital nursing unit, has always been considered essential to the effectiveness of the nursing unit. The HUC coordinates activities on the nursing unit, transcribes the doctors' orders, and usually functions under the direction of the nurse manager or unit manager. Everyone who works on or visits the nursing unit depends on the HUC for information and assistance (Fig. 1-1).

Comments often heard in the hospital include the following: "It's one of the most important positions on the nursing unit," "We are so disorganized if the HUC is not here," "The HUC creates the attitude for the entire unit," "The HUC sets the pace for the day's work," and "The health unit coordinators know everything." When walking onto a nursing unit, it is usually obvious if an efficient HUC is working on that unit. If the HUC is having a "bad day" or is in a "bad mood," the whole unit is affected because everyone has to interact with the HUC. It is important to maintain a positive, friendly attitude when one is working on the nursing unit. The HUC can enhance or inhibit the delivery of health care to patients on the nursing unit. The health unit coordinating practice may vary from hospital to hospital and from unit to unit; therefore, it is important for jobseekers to carefully read the HUC job description.

The role of the HUC has changed and expanded over the years, and the role is again changing and expanding with the introduction of electronic records and computer physician order entry.

History and Evolution

Similar to any other health profession, the position of HUC has evolved through four stages:
- On-the-job training
- Formal education

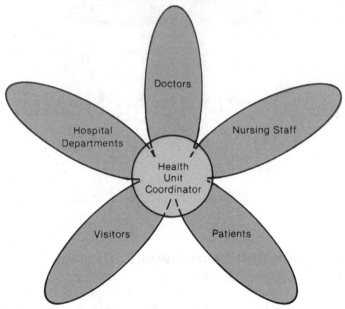

FIGURE 1-1 ▲ The HUC is responsible for coordinating the activities of nursing staff, doctors, hospital departments, patients, and visitors to the nursing unit.

- Formation of a national association
- Certification or licensure

On-the-Job Training

- **1940s**—The HUC profession started during World War II to compensate for the drastic shortage of nurses. "Floor secretaries" were trained on the job to assist the registered nurse with non-clinical tasks. On-the-job training continued through the early 1960s.

Formal Education

- **1966**—The first educational program for health unit coordinating was offered at a vocational school in Minneapolis. The title was changed to "ward clerk."
- **1970**—Ruth Stryker wrote one of the first textbooks for health unit coordinating, *The Hospital Ward Clerk*, which was published by C. V. Mosby.
- Today, before they are employed, most HUCs are educated at one of the many community colleges or vocational schools, or in a hospital-based program.

Formation of a National Association

- **1980**—The first organizational meeting was held in Phoenix, Arizona, on August 23, 1980; attendees were led by Myrna LaFleur in a

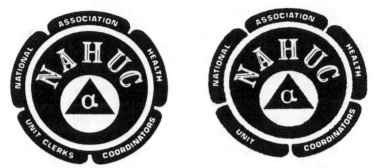

Logo prior to 1990   Logo as of 1990

FIGURE 1-2 ▲ The logo of the National Association of Health Unit Coordinators. The five outer segments represent doctors, nursing staff, patients, visitors, and hospital departments. The circle that connects these segments is symbolic of the role of the health unit coordinator (HUC) in coordinating the activities of the five groups.

discussion about forming a national association of HUCs. During this meeting, the founding members declared "health unit coordinator" as the chosen title for this profession and announced the formation of a national association for HUCs to be called the *National Association of Health Unit Coordinators/Clerks (NAHUC)*.

- **1982**—The first annual NAHUC convention was held in San Antonio, Texas.
- **1990**—The NAHUC dropped "Clerk" from its name, as is shown in Fig. 1-2, which depicts the organization's logo.
- **2006**—The 25th annual NAHUC convention was held in San Antonio, Texas.
- The NAHUC Standard of Practice and Code of Ethics may be found in Appendix F.

Five Reasons to Become a Member of the National Association of Health Unit Coordinators (NAHUC)

1. Professional representation
2. Format for sharing ideas and challenges—to be prepared and proactive regarding changes that are taking place in the HUC profession
3. National networking
4. National directory
5. Opportunity to develop leadership skills

Certification or Licensure

Certification is the process of testifying to or endorsing that a person has met certain standards. Passing the national certification examination indicates that one has met a standard of excellence and is competent to practice health unit coordinating.

- **1983**—The first national certification examination was offered.

This test is offered to anyone with a general education degree (GED) or a high school diploma. It is not necessary for those who take the test to be a member of the NAHUC or to have completed an educational program (some HUCs were trained on the job and have acquired years of experience).

Recertification

Certified HUCs must be recertified periodically to ensure that they stay current in their field of practice. Recertification may be achieved by taking the test every 3 years or by obtaining continuing education unit (CEU) hours. The NAHUC offers opportunities for obtaining CEUs, as do many employers.

Five Reasons to Become Certified

1. Enhanced credibility
2. Opportunity to gain a broader perspective of health unit coordinating (not just one specialty)—be prepared and proactive regarding changes that are taking place in the health unit coordinating profession
3. Increased mobility, geographically and vertically
4. Peer and public recognition and respect
5. Improved self-image

NAHUC and NAHUC Certification Information

To receive a National Association of Health Unit Coordinators (NAHUC) or certification test application, contact the NAHUC:

Phone: Toll-free: 1-888-22-NAHUC
Local: 815-633-4351
Mailing address: 1947 Madron Road
Rockford, IL 61107

Fax: 815-633-4438
E-mail: office@nahuc.org
Website: www.nahuc.org

Recent Changes Within the Health Care System

As technology continues to advance, the way health care is provided continues to change. Hospitals are moving toward a paperless system. Many hospitals have implemented the **electronic medical record**

(EMR) and the **computer physician order entry (CPOE)**. **Clinical decision support systems (CDSSs)** are computerized programs that provide to the physician, at the point of ordering, suggestions or default values for drug doses, routes, and frequencies. This program also may be used to perform such tasks as drug allergy checks, drug–laboratory value checks, and drug–drug interaction checks.

A patient's medication-related history is entered (by the patient's admitting nurse) into the system at the time of admission. When the physician is entering the patient's orders, the system provides prompts that warn against the possibility of drug interaction, allergy, or overdose. The system also may provide reminders to the physician regarding tasks such as ordering aspirin for a patient who is going home after having heart surgery. The CPOE can be remarkably effective in reducing the rate of serious medication errors. Studies conducted by the Leapfrog group have shown that the CPOE, if implemented in all urban hospitals in the United States, could prevent as many as 907,600 serious medication errors or adverse drug events (ADEs) each year. Studies have also shown that the EMR and CPOE reduce length of stay; reduce retests; reduce turn around times for laboratory, pharmacy, and radiology request; and deliver cost savings. This system, once in place nationally, will provide local, state, and federal governments with the data required to direct therapies, medical personnel, and supplies during an emergency.

The up-front cost of implementing CPOE use is a major obstacle for hospitals. Also, cultural obstacles may hinder CPOE implementation in that many physicians resist the idea of entering their orders via computer. Many hospitals have implemented the CPOE, but predictions suggest that it will take at least 5 years for the system to be implemented nationally.

The Impact of the EMR and the CPOE on the Role of the HUC

The responsibilities of the HUC change with the implementation of the EMR and the CPOE, allowing a greater focus on customer service. Most of the HUC's time has been spent on transcription of orders and paper chart management. Now, HUCs will have a more efficient role in traffic control, coordination of care, and management of the EMR. (See job description later.) Physician orders will be entered directly into the computer by the physician and automatically sent to the appropriate departments. Medication orders are automatically entered into the electronic medication administration record (E-MAR). The HUCs will no longer have to transcribe physicians' orders.

An HUC job description that incorporates implementation of the EMR and CPOE may include the following:
- Coordinate administrative functions on the nursing unit.
- Provide decision making and follow-up action to ensure effective communication and information flow throughout the nursing department.

- Perform receptionist/clerical duties on the nursing unit.
- Handle customer problems or collect necessary data and follow-through to the appropriate person for problem resolution.
- Monitor and maintain the EMR.
- Place requests for items from the Nutritional Care department and other unit supplies.
- Coordinate patient activities and patient information.
- Assist the nursing staff as needed with processing of medical records related to patient admission, discharge, and transfer.
- Maintain confidentiality of patient information.
- Integrate/scan into the EMR any paper documents created by caregivers.
- Send electronic requisitions for clerical, office, nutritional care, and medical supplies, and maintain adequate supply levels on the nursing unit.
- Input data for reports and assist in the coordination of mandatory education and assessment.
- Maintain the nursing bulletin board.
- Assist with staffing scheduling.
- Compile and prepare statistical data for reports.
- Provide assistance with process improvement.

Preparing for the Change to the EMR and the CPOE

Change is most often an opportunity for growth. Be proactive! Education is essential for attaining success with this changing technology. Communication and organizational skills are required for interfacing with health care personnel, visitors, and patients. The following are suggestions of ways to prepare for changes that are taking place in the HUC position:

- Complete an HUC program.
- Complete management classes related to health care.
- Attend in-services that are offered through the hospital or classes that are offered at local community colleges that relate to communication or related administrative skills.
- Complete computer classes to become efficient in or gain a working knowledge of advanced word processing and cultivate skills in database, spreadsheet, and e-mail functions (typing skills are essential).
- Become a member of the National Association of Health Unit Coordinators—receive the newsletter and attend the educational conferences.
- Become certified by taking the NAHUC certification test.

Career Paths

After acquiring experience and completing the required educational program, the HUC can advance to a management position. Possible management positions include those of health unit/service manager and health information manager. Employment information for both management positions is provided on the next page.

Possible Career Ladder Opportunities

(For more information about these positions and about community college programs that offer degree programs and classes for these positions, the titles may be searched on the Internet.)

Health Unit/Service Manager (also called *Health Care Administrator*)

Education Requirement

A Master's degree is the standard credential, although a Bachelor's degree is adequate for some entry level positions in smaller facilities and in health information management.

Responsibilities

Plan, direct, coordinate, and supervise the delivery of health care—provide leadership in a variety of health service and business office settings. Responsibilities include directing others, coordinating work activities, monitoring financial resources, and helping staff to develop an effective organization.

Medical and health service managers include specialists (in charge of specific clinical departments or services) and generalists (manage or help manage an entire facility or system).

Work Environment

Most medical or health service managers work in facilities such as hospitals, nursing care facilities, and group practices. Some managers have their own offices; others share an office with other managers or staff. Some managers oversee more than one health care facility. The hours are long.

Job Outlook

Employment for health service managers is expected to grow faster than average as technology advances and health care expands.

Health Information Managers

Education Requirement

A bachelor's degree from an accredited program and a Registered Health Information Administrator (RHIA) certification from the American Health Information Management Association is required.

Responsibilities

The HUC is responsible for the maintenance and security of all patient EMRs. The health service manager must keep up with current computer and software technology and legislative requirements and developments regarding maintenance and security of the patient EMR.

(Continued)

Possible Career Ladder Opportunities—Cont'd

Work Environment

Health information managers work in health care settings such as hospitals, nursing homes, home health care agencies, and health maintenance organizations.

Job Outlook

Rapid employment growth is projected with implementation of the EMR.

Summary

Health unit coordinating is a recognized health care profession. Individuals who practice as HUCs soon realize that they have far-reaching effects on the delivery of health care to patients. This job is changing, and although change can be stressful, it also can be exciting and can result in opportunities for growth. Implementation of the EMR is currently expanding the administrative and management roles of the HUC.

CHAPTER 2

Ensuring Effective Interpersonal Communication

Expanding Communication Role

The health unit coordinator (HUC) is the liaison between the doctor, the nursing staff, ancillary departments, visitors, and patients. Communication is the main function of the HUC, and with the implementation of the electronic medical record (EMR), this role is expanding. Often, the HUC assists doctors, nurses, and ancillary personnel in use of the computer system. The HUC has a larger role in listening to visitor, patient, and nursing unit personnel complaints and in problem solving. Working in the health care environment can become extremely stressful at times. If communication breaks down and tempers become short, chaos most likely will result, and the risk of error will be increased. It is important for the HUC to know how to deal with and ease the tension to maintain the efficiency of the unit.

Communication Skills

Most of us spend much of our time communicating, but few of us communicate as effectively as we should. Many factors contribute to communication difficulties. For instance, the English language has grown considerably throughout its history, and the language comprises approximately 750,000 words. It is impossible to know how many words an individual may have in their vocabulary, but it is believed that the average educated person comprehends about 20,000 words. The medical world also has a growing language of its own that is made up of abbreviations and medical terms. Some words have more than one meaning. For instance, a *chip* in the computer world has a much different meaning than a *chip* used in a poker game.

Communication is 55% visual (facial and body language, symbolism), 38% vocal (qualities such as tone, loudness, firmness, hesitations, and pauses), and 7% verbal (actual words) (Fig. 2-1). Inconsistency is often apparent between what a person is saying and how they appear.

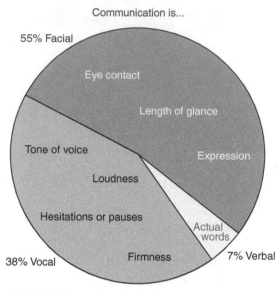

FIGURE 2-1 ▲ Verbal and nonverbal communication.

("Of course I'm listening to you, Mother," says the 9-year-old boy as he sits glued to the television set, leaving the mother wondering whether the child is indeed listening to her.)

Another major weakness in the communication process involves poor listening skills. Often, we are thinking of something else while the speaker is talking to us; we may be formulating a response or prejudging what is being said.

Any communication consists of the following:

- A **sender**—the person who transmits the message
- A **message**—the images, feelings, and ideas transmitted
- A **receiver**—the person who receives the message
- **Feedback**—the response to the message

For communication to be effective, both the sender and the receiver must be actively involved in communicating with one another. The sender must translate mental images, feelings, and ideas into symbols to communicate them to the receiver. This process is called *encoding.* **Encoding** involves the decision of the sender about whether to send the message through verbal or nonverbal symbols. What are the right words to use so the receiver will understand the message? What is the proper inflection? What body language and eye signals can enhance the words? When the idea, feeling, or image is encoded, complete with nonverbal cues, it becomes a message.

As the message reaches the receiver, the verbal and nonverbal symbols are decoded. **Decoding** is the process of translating the symbols received from the sender to determine the message. Unsuccessful decoding can be caused by inconsistency in the verbal and nonverbal symbols received

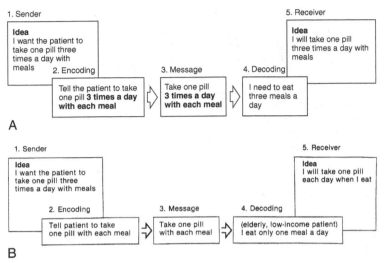

FIGURE 2-2 ▲ **A,** An example of successful communication. **B,** An example of unsuccessful communication.

from the sender (Fig. 2-2, *A, B*). Differences between the sender and the receiver in terms of lifestyle, age, cultural background, or environment, along with poor listening habits on the part of the receiver, are other reasons for incorrect decoding.

Verbal and Nonverbal Communication

Verbal communication is the use of language or the actual words spoken, whereas nonverbal communication is the use of eye contact, body language, facial expression, or symbolic expressions such as clothing that communicate a message. Sometimes, verbal and nonverbal communications contradict each other.

Nonverbal communication can be separated further into two types: symbolic and body language.

Nonverbal Language	
Symbolic	**Body Language**
Clothing	Posture
Hair	Ambulation
Jewelry	Touching
Body art	Personal distance
Cosmetics	Eye contact
Automobile	Breathing
House	Hand gestures
Perfume or cologne	Facial expressions

Listening

As described by Dr. Stephen R. Covey in his best-selling book, *Seven Habits of Highly Effective People*, listening occurs at five different levels, depending on the interest in what is being said or what else is being done while the individual is listening.

The five levels of listening are:
1. **Ignoring**—making no effort to listen
2. **Pretend listening**—giving the appearance that one is listening
3. **Selective listening**—hearing only the parts that interest one
4. **Attentive listening (also called *active listening*)**—paying attention to and focusing on what the speaker says, and comparing this with one's own experience
5. **Empathetic listening**—listening and responding with both the heart and the mind to truly understand; realizing that every person has a right to feel as they do

Guidelines for Improving Listening Skills
- Stop talking.
- Teach yourself to concentrate (attentive listening).
- Take time to listen.
- Listen with your eyes (practice empathetic listening by looking into the sender's eyes).
- Listen to what is being said, not only to how it is being said (use both attentive and empathic listening).
- Suspend judgment.
- Do not interrupt the speaker.
- Remove distractions.
- Listen for both feeling and content (seek to understand).

Feedback

Feedback, the response to a message that is sent, is the final component of the communication process. Effective communication is virtually impossible without it. Feedback tells the sender how much of the message was understood, indicates whether the receiver agrees or disagrees with the message, and helps the sender correct confusing or vague language.

Feedback can be given as a nod, an answer to a question, or a more detailed response that encourages further communication and assists the sender in developing ideas or sharing feelings.

Guidelines for Improving Feedback Skills
- Use paraphrasing (repeat the message to the sender in one's own words).
- Repeat the last word or words of the message.
- Use specific rather than general feedback.
- Use constructive rather than destructive feedback.
- Do not deny the sender's feelings.

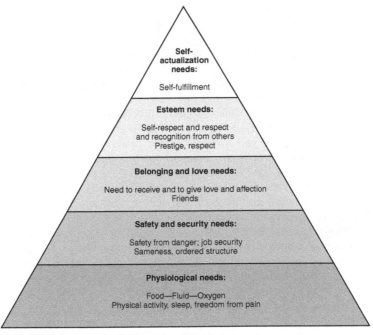

FIGURE 2–3 ▲ Maslow's Hierarchy of Needs.

To develop effective communication and interpersonal skills, one must first gain an understanding of interpersonal behavior. A model used in this chapter to explain human behavior is Maslow's Hierarchy of Needs (Fig. 2-3), which was developed by the late Abraham Maslow, a famous psychologist. Maslow's Hierarchy of Needs emphasizes that all people have the same basic needs and that these needs motivate and influence a person's behavior either consciously or unconsciously.

The needs are arranged in a pyramid with the most basic or immediate needs at the bottom of the pyramid and the less critical needs at the top. The lower the need is in the pyramid, the more influence it has on a person's behavior. By looking at the pyramid, one can see that these needs may be related to the hospitalized patient, and in this way, their behavior may be better understood (e.g., being "nothing by mouth" [NPO] for a test, not receiving visitation from family members).

Intercultural Communication Skills

The United States often is referred to as a "melting pot" because of the multitude of cultures that have been blended into the American culture. Cultures are formed when groups of people spend an extended time together. Each of us has values, beliefs, habits, and customs that result from our cultural backgrounds. Subcultures are made up of smaller groups of people within the larger culture who have common ethnic, occupational, religious, or physical characteristics (e.g., within the American culture, subcultures include the elderly, teens, nurses, Christians, and athletes, among others).

It is essential for health care workers to understand and evaluate their values, beliefs, and customs before they work with and care for people whose cultures differ from their own. Many conflicts that occur in the health care delivery system are caused by cultural misunderstandings (e.g., verbal or nonverbal language, lack of courtesy, objectivity vs. subjectivity). Providing culturally sensitive care involves taking the time to learn about the cultural backgrounds of patients and may involve incorporating their beliefs and practices into their care. Often, people judge others by comparing the values and beliefs of individuals with their own and find it difficult to accept other cultures. This is referred to as *ethnocentrism*.

The HUC may have attitudes regarding a patient who refuses treatment because of religious beliefs, a patient who is admitted for sex-change surgery, or a patient who is a substance abuser, just to name a few examples of possible cultural conflicts. These attitudes must not be allowed to affect the quality of care given to these patients.

HUCs, similar to all health care providers, must be aware of their own cultural biases and must avoid stereotyping others as the result of assumptions or conclusions drawn about a patient or a coworker that are based on race, ethnicity, or other factors. All patients and coworkers deserve to be treated and respected as unique individuals regardless of their gender, age, economic status, religion, sexual orientation, educational level, occupation, physical makeup or limitations, or command of the English language. Often, when we are speaking to someone from a different culture who does not speak English well, our attitudes and feelings are evident. The following guidelines will assist the individual in this process.

Guidelines for Speaking to Someone Who Does Not Speak English Well

- Do not shout.
- Talk distinctly and slowly.
- Emphasize key words.
- Let the listener read your lips.
- Use printed words and pictures.
- Do not use slang or jargon.
- Organize your thoughts.
- Choose your words carefully.
- Construct your sentences to say exactly what you want to say.
- Observe body language carefully.
- Try to pronounce names correctly.
- Ask for feedback to assess understanding.

Assertiveness

Have you ever said yes to a request when you really wanted to say no, or left a conversation wishing you had "stood up for yourself"? If your answer is yes, then you responded in a **nonassertive behavioral style.**

Have you ever allowed a situation to get out of control, then "blown up," and later wished you had handled the situation better? If your answer is yes, then you responded in an **aggressive behavioral style.**

In a middle ground, third type of response, an **assertive behavioral style,** an individual expresses their wants and desires in an honest and appropriate way, while respecting the rights of other people.

As an HUC, you may have to ask patients or visitors to change their behavior to conform to regulations and rules, or to allow for the comfort of others. Knowing you have a choice of behavioral styles and choosing the right way to handle a given situation will help you to communicate more effectively (Table 2-1).

Assertiveness Skills

The goal of using assertiveness in communication is to arrive at an **"I win, you win"** conclusion—a workable compromise. A workable compromise is a solution to a conflict that is satisfactory to all involved parties. Four assertiveness skills that may be used to reach a workable compromise are broken record, fogging, negative assertion, and negative inquiry.

Broken Record

The broken record is an assertiveness skill that allows you to say "no" over and over again without raising your voice or getting irritated or angry. You must be persistent and not give reasons, excuses, or explanations for not doing what the other person wants you to do. By doing this, you can ignore manipulative traps and argumentative baiting.

Fogging

Fogging allows you to accept manipulative criticism and anxiety-producing statements by offering no resistance and using a noncommittal reply, acknowledging that there may be some truth in what the critic is saying, yet retaining the right to remain your own judge. Fogging makes it hard for the other person to understand exactly what you are saying.

Negative Assertion

Negative assertion allows you to accept errors and faults without becoming defensive or angry. It is a technique of admitting errors without letting them affect your perception of your worth as a human being. It includes not using self-deprecating statements like "That was so stupid of me."

TABLE 2-1	Comparison of Nonassertive, Aggressive, and Assertive Behavioral Styles		
Components	**Nonassertive**	**Aggressive**	**Assertive**
Rights	Does not stand up for rights	Stands up for rights but violates the rights of others	Stands up for rights without violating the rights of others
Choice	Allows others to choose (to avoid conflict)	Chooses for others	Chooses for self
Belief	I'm not OK, you're OK; lose/win	I'm OK, you're not OK; win/lose	I'm OK, you're OK; win/win
Responsibility	Others responsible for behavior Blames himself for poor results; may blame others for feelings	Responsible for others' behavior Blames others for poor results Feelings aren't important	Responsible for own behavior Assumes responsibility for own errors; assumes responsibility for feelings
Traits	Self-denying, apologetic, timid, emotionally dishonest, has difficulty saying "no," guilty, whining, "poor me"	Dominates, humiliates, uses sarcasm Self-enhancing at the expense of others, opinionated	Expresses feelings, feels good about self, candid, diplomatic, listens, eye contact
Goals	Does not achieve goals	Achieves goals at the expense of others	May achieve goals
Word choices	Minimizing words such as "I'm sorry," "I believe," "I think," "Little," and "sort of" General instead of specific statements; statements disguised as questions	"You" statements Always/never statements Demands instead of requests	"I understand..." "I feel..." "I apologize..." Neutral language Concise statements
Body language	Lack of eye contact; slumping, downtrodden posture; words and nonverbal messages that don't match	"Looking-through-you" eye contact; tense, impatient posture	Erect, relaxed posture; eye contact; verbal and nonverbal messages match

Negative Inquiry

Negative inquiry allows you to actively prompt criticism by asking questions to use the information or, if manipulative, to exhaust it. By doing this, you obtain clarification about the criticism and may succeed in bringing out possible hidden issues that may really be the point.

Dealing With an Angry Telephone Caller

The HUC may be confronted by an angry or disgruntled telephone caller. These steps should help you handle the situation effectively:

- When answering the telephone, always identify yourself by nursing unit, name, and status. Doing this puts one on a more personal level with the caller. Also, a caller may become more upset if it is necessary for them to ask questions to find out who you are.
- Avoid putting the person on hold. Placing an angry person on hold often escalates their anger.
- Listen to what the caller is saying. Do not become defensive. Keep in mind that the caller is not angry with you personally.
- Write down what the caller is saying. The notes may come in handy, and focusing on taking notes can help you control your anger.
- Acknowledge the anger. Use phrases such as, "I understand that you are angry," and "I hear your frustration."
- Do not allow the caller to become abusive. Say, "I feel you are becoming abusive," or "Please call me back in a few minutes so we can talk about this calmly."

Using Communication and Interpersonal Skills in the Health Care Setting

The HUC may use communication and interpersonal skills in daily work in five major ways:

1. **Obtaining information**—Often, you must obtain information to communicate in a correct and timely manner. Apply assertiveness skills to ask a question correctly, use appropriate listening skills when receiving the response, and use the guidelines for speaking to a person who does not speak English well.

2. **Providing information**—The HUC provides information to visitors, doctors, nursing staff, and other hospital departments, as well as to institutions outside the hospital. Being aware of verbal and nonverbal use of language is helpful when one is doing this.

3. **Developing trust**—Trust is vital to a healthy work environment, and assertive communication plays a big role in establishing and maintaining trust.

4. **Showing understanding**—An understanding of the needs of patients, families, and coworkers in the context of Maslow's Hierarchy of Needs can foster successful communication in the work environment.

5. Relieving stress—Stress in the workplace is a constant; how you manage it makes a difference. Recognizing the three behavioral types and using assertiveness skills can be helpful in this area. Use of effective listening skills may help you to avoid, or may alleviate, stressful situations.

Precepting Sudents/New Employees

When given the opportunity to precept (to train or instruct) a student or to orient a new employee to the nursing unit/hospital, you should keep in mind what it was like to begin a new job and to be inexperienced—were you made to feel welcome, or were you made to feel that you were in the way? How did this affect your clinical/orientation experience? When you are selected to be a preceptor (trainer or teacher), your nurse manager is demonstrating confidence in your expertise and in your knowledge and ability to teach the student or new employee what they need to know.

To provide the best learning experience, it is important for you to make new employees feel comfortable so they will ask questions, if necessary, to gain a full understanding of what you are teaching. Each person learns at a different pace; some will remember what you have told them the first time, some will need to write it down, and others will need to actually perform the task before they master it. The following guidelines should assist you in becoming an efficient preceptor and in providing a successful clinical experience or orientation.

Guidelines for the HUC Preceptor

- Provide a copy of dates and times the student or new employee is to be on the nursing unit to complete their clinical experience (provide a copy of your schedule to the student and the student's instructor or to the new employee).
- Obtain a list of objectives (provided by the hospital or by the school), so all are clear on what is to be accomplished by the end of the clinical experience.
- Take students/new employees on a tour of the nursing unit and hospital, so they can become aware of where restrooms, cafeteria, and hospital departments are located.
- Set a positive example—be on time each day, return on time from appropriate breaks, and maintain a positive attitude regarding your job, the hospital, the administration, and nursing unit personnel.
- If the student/new employee does not call before being tardy or absent, it is the preceptor's responsibility to notify the instructor and/or the appropriate nurse manager.
- Notify the student or the new employee and staffing if you are going to be tardy or absent, or if you transferred to another unit (preferably an hour before the start of the shift).

- Stay with the student/new employee to monitor progress, and check off objectives as completed with competence, as instructed in the clinical/orientation packet.
- Provide feedback to the student/new employee, and offer suggestions for improvement.
- Notify the student's instructor and/or the new employee's nurse manager if the student/new employee is not dressed according to hospital/school dress code (the student may have a more strict dress code), is not performing in an appropriate and professional manner, or is having difficulty completing objectives.
- Notify the student's instructor or the new employee's nurse manager if you have questions or concerns.
- Notify the student's instructor or the new employee's nurse manager immediately if you have serious concerns.
- Complete an evaluation form regarding the student's clinical experience.

Guidelines for the HUC Student or New Employee

- Be sure you know when and where you are to complete your clinical experience, and know the name of your preceptor.
- If you are a student, provide your preceptor with a list of objectives and the instructor's telephone and/or pager number.
- The student/new employee should notify the nursing unit, the preceptor, and the instructor or nurse manager an hour before the start of the shift (unless emergency) if they are going to be tardy or absent.
- The student must notify the instructor if they leave the hospital before the end of the shift.
- It is the student's responsibility to notify their instructor if the preceptor is going to be late, absent, or is transferred to another unit.
- The student or new employee should arrive dressed appropriately and prepared to learn and work each day, and should be accountable for completing the required learning objectives.
- The student needs to be flexible and should refrain from saying, "That's not the way we were taught in class" or "That's not the way we did it at Previous Community Hospital."
- The student or new employee should communicate openly with the preceptor and instructor or nurse manager regarding any problems with their clinical performance.
- The student/new employee should have the list of objectives/ evaluation forms completed and signed off by the preceptor 2 days before the last clinical day.
- The student/new employee should complete an evaluation form regarding their clinical experience or orientation.

Managing Patient Activities and Information

Webster's Dictionary defines *manage* as "to control or guide." The HUC who learns to "manage or guide" certain facets within their job is able to realize the full potential of health unit coordinating. The HUC is responsible for managing patient activities and information. A census worksheet is a tool that can help one accomplish this task efficiently. It includes each patient's name, room, and bed number and provides blank spaces in which one can record pertinent data. Maintaining an up-to-date census worksheet allows the HUC to quickly answer questions frequently asked by doctors, health care personnel, and visitors about patients. To use a census worksheet effectively, follow these guidelines:

- Print a census worksheet at the beginning of the shift.
- Record patient activities that pertain to duties that the HUC would perform, such as scheduled diagnostic procedures, surgeries, planned discharges, transfers, etc.
- Note the scheduled time of each patient activity.
- Record the time the patient leaves the unit, their destination, and the time they return.
- List any other important information (e.g., DNR orders, visitor and phone call guidelines, NINP, isolation status).
- Tape the census worksheet to the desktop (near the telephone) for easy reference.
- Update the census worksheet throughout the shift.

Continuous Quality Improvement

Continuous quality improvement (CQI), a requirement of the Joint Commission (TJC), is the practice of continuously improving quality at every level of every department for every function of the health care organization. Most hospitals have CQI committees that oversee the assessment and improvement of work processes, in addition to focusing on what patients want and need. The quality movement is global because CQI results in products and services of better quality. Competition to provide the best product and service in the most efficient manner has increased worldwide. The HUC is often asked to serve on a committee to solve quality improvement problems related to nursing unit clerical processes. A committee assigned this process may use two techniques: application of the following problem-solving model and brainstorming.

The Five-Step Problem-Solving Model

1. Identify and analyze the problem.
2. Identify alternative plans for the solution.
3. Choose the best plan.
4. Put the plan for solution in place.
5. Evaluate the plan after it has been in place for a given time.

Brainstorming is a structured group activity that allows 3 to 10 people to tap into the creativity of the group to identify new ideas. Typically used in quality improvement efforts, the technique is designed to reveal probable causes of, and possible solutions for, quality problems.

Summary

Effective communication is essential in the health care setting. Quality patient care requires an efficient, professional, and culturally sensitive team. Health care can be extremely stressful, so it is vital that personnel remain calm, exercise assertiveness skills, and have empathy for patients and coworkers. Each member of a health care team is important and necessary, and it is imperative that staff members maintain a positive attitude regarding the job, hospital, administration, and nursing unit personnel. About one third of your time is spent at your job!

CHAPTER 3

Using Communication Devices

Communicating and operating communication devices are among the most important responsibilities of the health unit coordinator (HUC) (Fig. 3-1). Implementation of the electronic medical record (EMR) has made it necessary for doctors, nurses, ancillary personnel, and HUCs to be better educated in computer technology (Fig. 3-1).

Telephone Etiquette

Speaking on the telephone requires a different type of interaction than speaking face-to-face. A good attitude toward telephone transactions and the use of proper telephone etiquette are essential for positive customer relations. Each time the telephone is used for communication, an image is created for the caller about the nursing unit and/or the hospital. Realize this, and handle each telephone conversation with care.

- Answer the telephone promptly and kindly, preferably before the third ring. If you are engaged in a conversation at the nurses' station, excuse yourself to answer the telephone.
- Identify yourself properly by stating location, name, and status, for example, "4 East, Stacey, Health Unit Coordinator." The manner in which you identify yourself and address the caller is the caller's first clue about your professional identity, self-esteem, mood, expectations, and willingness to continue the communication. At this time, you are conveying to the caller an image of the hospital. When you identify yourself correctly, the caller is saved time and confusion is eliminated.
- Speak into the telephone—make sure the mouthpiece is not under your chin; this would make it difficult for the caller to hear.
- Give the caller your undivided attention—it is difficult to focus on the telephone conversation while you are attempting to do something else.

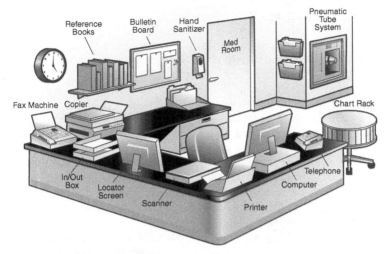

FIGURE 3-1 ▲ The HUC's work area is the nurses' station. Communication devices are within easy reach.

- Speak clearly and distinctly—do not eat food or chew gum while you are talking on the telephone.
- Always be courteous—say "Please" and "Thank you."
- When you do not know the answer, state that you will locate someone who can help the caller.
- If it is necessary to step away or answer another call, place the caller on hold after you have asked permission to do so and have waited for an answer, for example, "May I put you on hold, Mr. Phillips, so I can find Jane to speak with you?"

Uses of the Hold Button

- Locate information or a person for the caller. Always return to the person on hold every 30 to 60 seconds—ask if they wish to remain on hold or if they would prefer to leave a return call number.
- Answer other phone lines. Return to the first caller after asking the second caller if they would hold or would like to leave a number to be called back.
- Protect patient confidentiality. Conversations held in the nursing station often involve confidential patient information and should not be overheard.

Taking Messages

When taking telephone messages, be sure to obtain all the information needed for the person for whom the call is intended, including the following:

- Who the message is for
- The caller's name

- The date and time of the call
- The purpose of the call
- The number to call back, if a return call is expected

Always write the information down. Always have a pad and pencil or pen near each telephone. Sign and deliver messages promptly.

Placing Telephone Calls

When you are asked to place a call to a doctor, to another department, or to someone outside the health care facility, make sure to plan the call as follows:

- If the call will be made to discuss a patient, have the patient's chart handy so that facts will be available when questions are asked. Also, write down the main facts that are to be discussed and the telephone number to be called if the line is busy and the call must be made later.
- Anyone who requests that a call be placed to discuss a patient should provide the patient's name and the reason for the call.
- Before you place a call for a nurse to a doctor, alert the nurse that the call is being placed, and ask the person who requested it to stay on the unit, if possible, or to designate someone else to take the call in their place.

Voice Mail

Voice mail is used in health care facilities, physicians' offices, and homes to receive incoming calls. To use voice mail effectively, follow the guidelines provided here.

- After listening to the recorded greeting and indicated tone, do the following:
  - Speak slowly and distinctly, so the person who is listening to the message can hear and understand what is being communicated.
  - If you are leaving a message, include the name of the patient and/or the doctor. Give the first and last names, and spell the last name.
  - If the message includes a telephone number or laboratory values, speak slowly and repeat the numbers twice, allowing time for the listener to record the information.
  - Always leave your name and telephone number, and repeat both twice (at the beginning of the message and at the end of the message) so the listener can call for clarification if necessary.

Telephone Directories

Most health care facilities have computer access to the doctors' roster that contains information, such as the following:

- Doctors who have admitting or visiting privileges (in alphabetical order)
- Each doctor's medical specialty

- Each doctor's office telephone number and answering service telephone number, if different

  When you are placing a telephone call, select the doctor's number with care because several doctors with the same name are often listed. If two doctors have the same first and last names, refer to their specialty to select the correct telephone number.

  Directories of extension numbers for hospital departments and pager numbers for key personnel are also available.

Locator System

Locators are small devices that are worn by nursing unit personnel, including HUCs (clipped on uniforms).

- A screen displays a list of the nursing unit personnel who wear the locators, along with their locations.
- If the locator is flipped over or obstructed, it may not show the nurse's location.
- The locator system is used for communication between nursing unit personnel and the nursing station.
- If the person who is wearing the locator needs help, a button on the locator may be pushed to call the nursing station.
- The HUC may call into a patient's room to speak to the nurse.
- This system is very helpful when personnel are covering more than one unit or are working as a "SWAT," meaning "on call for all units in the hospital." (Some hospitals use pagers or cell phones for this purpose.)

Pocket Pagers

When you are using a voice pager, dial the pager number and state the message. Always repeat the entire message twice, including the name of the person who is being paged and the extension number that they are to call.

When you use a digital pager, dial the pager number and enter the number the person is to call. Wait at least 5 minutes before paging a second time, unless the situation is stat. Some nursing units use a number code that is entered at the end of the call-back number—with number 1 indicating stat, number 2 indicating as soon as possible, and number 3 indicating at the individual's convenience.

Unit Intercom Etiquette

Always identify yourself and your location when you are answering a patient's call light. When two or more patients are staying in the room, ask the patient to state their name.

The intercom also may be used to locate nursing personnel if locators or individual pagers are not used. To page personnel on the intercom, depress the button that allows the message to be heard in each of the rooms.

A simple message such as "Susan, please call the nurses' station" is all that is needed.

Be selective about the information communicated over the intercom because some types of messages may prove embarrassing to the patient. Keep messages as brief as possible, and do not communicate any confidential patient information to a nurse over the intercom.

Voice (Overhead) Paging System

The voice paging system is a system by which the hospital switchboard operator, upon request, pages someone on a speaker that is heard in every area of the hospital. To locate a doctor with this system, you should dial the hospital switchboard operator, provide the name of the doctor who is needed, and give the telephone extension number the doctor is to call when located. The operator announces the name of the doctor who is needed and relays the message.

The operator also uses the voice paging system to locate a doctor regarding calls received from outside the hospital. Doctors will often ask the HUC to listen for their page, especially when they are in a patient's room. When a page for a doctor is announced, you should contact the operator for the message and relay it to the doctor.

Copiers and Shredders

- Many nursing units have a photocopy machine available for making copies of written or typed materials.
- The fax machine also can be used to make a minimum number of copies.
- Never copy patient records unless there is a written physician's order to do so.
- Patient forms that contain confidential information cannot be thrown in the wastebasket.
- Shredder machines or containers for material to be picked up and taken to be shredded are placed on nursing units.
- Chart forms with labels with patient names and identification numbers that do not have documentation on them must be shredded when discarded.

Fax Machine

- Reports and other documents are faxed to and from health care institutions and doctors' offices.
- In hospitals that have not implemented the EMR, doctors' order sheets are faxed to the pharmacy.
- When doctors' orders are faxed, the fax machine may be used to make a copy of the orders to give to the appropriate nurse. If the health care facility has implemented computer physician order

entry (CPOE), this would not be necessary because the orders would be entered into the computer by the doctor and would be sent to the pharmacy automatically.

- Fax machines have a redial option that allows a document to be sent to the location last programmed into the machine. Because many health care workers use the fax machine, the redial option should not be used; doing so may cause a document to be sent to the wrong location.

Pneumatic Tube

- Do not place specimens obtained through a painful procedure (e.g., cerebrospinal fluid [CSF], bone marrow) into the pneumatic tube.
- When a tube that is carrying supplies or other items arrives at the nursing unit, it is the responsibility of the HUC to remove the tube from the pneumatic tube system as soon as possible and disperse the items appropriately.
- Some health care facilities have a telelift system that is operated in much the same way and for the same purposes as the tube system. It consists of a small boxcar that is carried on a conveyor belt to designated locations. A keypad is used to program the car to go to a specific unit or department.

Computers

- The health care facility's computer system contains a great deal of information that is confidential and must not be tampered with; therefore, a security system is used.
- When hired, each employee is assigned an identification code and a password.
- When the computer is used, a password is required to gain entry into the system.
- Employees are asked to sign a confidentiality statement. One should never share their identification code and password with anyone.
- It is imperative for patient confidentiality and employee protection that employees sign off of the computer when leaving the nursing unit for a break, or when going home.
- When someone is signed onto the computer with their personal identification code, any misuse will be tracked back to that individual.

E-mail

E-mail (electronic mail) is used to send and receive messages and frequently is used for communication between the HUC and hospital personnel and departments within the hospital.

Guidelines to be followed when e-mail is used in the workplace include the following:
- Do not use for personal messages or to send inappropriate material such as jokes.
- Send or respond to the necessary person or department only; refrain from "sending to all" or using "reply to all" unless necessary.

Computer Use in Hospitals in Which the Paper Patient Chart Is Used

Most hospitals provide several computer terminals on each nursing unit so that doctors, residents, and nursing staff members have easy access to patient information such as patient location, diagnostic test results, and physicians' orders. The HUC usually has a separate terminal for placing orders and entering discharges, transfers, and admissions. Many health care facilities have bedside computers available in each patient's room on which nursing personnel can record care and treatments performed. These records generally are printed every 24 hours for placement on the patient's paper chart. At times, the computer is shut down for scheduled routine servicing (usually at night) or because of mechanical failure. During these times, downtime requisitions are used to process information. When computer function returns, the information processed by the paper method must be entered into the computer.

Computer Use in Hospitals With the EMR c̄ CPOE

When the EMR c̄ CPOE is implemented, the HUC usually has a separate work area that includes a desktop computer. Multiple desktop computers are available for doctors, nurses, and authorized health care workers to use (Fig. 3-2). Computers on wheels (COWs) and tablet computers that may be used at the patient's bedside are also provided for nurses or doctors to use. Many nurses use personal data processors, which are handheld computers into which software, such as a nurses' drug reference, a medical dictionary, and other nursing reference books, has been downloaded. Nurses use this information to calculate drug dosages and gather research information.

The doctor can enter orders directly into the patient's EMR and access computerized reports, diagnostic images, diagnostic test results, and nurses' notes for review. Nurses can enter documentation and notes directly into the patient's medical record and can access doctors' orders, diagnostic test results, diagnostic images for evaluation, and computerized reports.

The HUC monitors the patient's EMR for required HUC tasks. A telephone icon appears on the computer screen next to the patient's name when an HUC task must be performed to complete the doctors' order. These tasks may include a telephone call to schedule a consult, a call placed to obtain medical records from another facility, and other tasks.

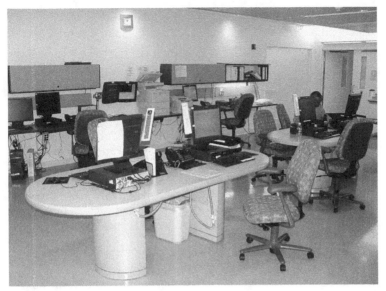

FIGURE 3–2 ▲ Computer stations on the nusing unit.

The HUC uses the computer to access doctors' telephone numbers and locate patients for visitors or doctors as needed. If requested to do so, the HUC enters data into the computer and may access computerized reports.

Document Scanner

A document scanner is a device that is used to transmit images of documents/pictures into a computer system (or set of computer programs) that is used to track and store electronic documents and/or images of paper documents.

- The document management system (DMS) uses bar codes to identify types of documents.
- The scanner is used by the HUC to scan outside documents, handwritten progress notes, reports, and other documents into the patient's EMR.
- These documents are sent to the health information management service (HIMS) and are certified by the health information technician before they become part of the patient's permanent EMR.
- Bundles of up to 14 documents may be placed in the scanner at a time, although documents that contain color (i.e., electrocardiograms) must be scanned alone.
- After documents have been scanned, the originals must be rubber-banded and placed in a bin to be picked up by someone from the HIMS department. These documents then are stored for a specified length of time before they are shredded.

Label Printer

A label printer (located near the HUC) is a machine that prints patient labels from information entered into the computer (these are placed on documents and items for identification purposes). Imprinter machines and imprinter cards are used in some facilities.

Nursing Unit Census Boards

The census board shows unit room numbers, admitting doctors' names, and the names of nurses assigned to all patients. Patient names may be omitted intentionally to maintain patient confidentiality. The HUC is assigned the responsibility of removing the names of discharged or transferred patients and adding the names of newly admitted or transferred patients. New Health Insurance Portability and Accountability Act (HIPAA) laws may change the current usage of census boards.

Nursing Unit Bulletin Board

The HUC may be assigned the responsibility of maintaining the nursing unit bulletin board. This responsibility involves posting material in an attractive manner and keeping the posted material current.

If the date were not indicated on the bulletin, the HUC would indicate the date posted. Policy changes are very important. It may be requested that each person should initial the notice after reading it, so the nurse manager will know that all unit employees have read it. The HUC then would place the initialed notice on the nurse manager's desk when it has been removed from the bulletin board. A neat board with up-to-date notices prompts unit personnel to read what is posted.

Summary

The ability of the HUC to use the computer, telephone, intercom, and other communication devices efficiently and effectively contributes to the smooth operation of the nursing unit. As technology advances, enhanced computer skills are becoming a necessity for the HUC. Accuracy in taking telephone messages and communicating them to the correct person is also necessary if a nursing unit is to be run efficiently.

CHAPTER 4

Management Techniques/Maintaining the Patient's Paper Chart and Electronic Medical Record

Prioritization

Management requires the ability to determine which task takes priority over another. A task that is usually of lower priority sometimes becomes a high-priority task. For example, filing or scanning a report into a patient's chart may become a matter of high priority if that patient is scheduled for surgery within a short time. Some tasks, such as ordering stat laboratory tests while conveying a message to the nurse about a patient who is returning from surgery, can be performed simultaneously.

The usual priority order of tasks is as follows:

1. Orders involving a patient in a medical crisis (takes priority over all other tasks)
2. Transcribing stat orders
3. Answering the nursing unit telephone (preferably before the third ring)
4. Communicating a telephoned message to the nurse that a patient has to be prepared to go to surgery, is now out of surgery and in the recovery room, or is returning to their room from surgery
5. Notifying the patient's nurse and doctor of stat laboratory results
6. Transcribing preop and postop orders
7. Transcribing new admission orders and daily routine orders
8. Transcribing discharge and transfer orders, so that clerical work can be processed by the time the patient is ready to leave or be transferred
9. Performing additional and routine tasks

✐ *TAKE NOTE*

When the electronic medical record (EMR) c̄ computer physician order entry (CPOE) has been implemented, the health unit coordinator (HUC) will not be transcribing patients' orders.

(Continued)

🖉 TAKE NOTE—Cont'd

Monitoring the EMR for HUC tasks will be a high priority. An icon (e.g., a telephone) usually is used to indicate an HUC task on the computer unit screen that contains the list of patients (census). HUC tasks may include scheduling procedures, placing phone calls, obtaining medical records from another facility, printing discharge instructions and prescriptions, scanning documents into the patient's EMR, and so forth. Otherwise, the priorities are the same.

It is important to constantly monitor the list of patients on the nursing unit for tasks. If tasks are missed or delayed, this could delay patients' diagnostic testing and/or treatment.

The following techniques may assist the HUC in managing the workload:

1. Ask for assistance when necessary.
2. Upon returning to the nursing unit from a break and finding several charts lying about, check each chart for new orders, place in the chart rack those that do not have new orders, read all new orders, notify the patient's nurse of any stats and provide the nurse with a copy of the orders, and fax or send copies to the pharmacy; then, proceed to transcribe all other orders, one chart at a time. If CPOE has been implemented, check the computer for tasks.
3. Always finish transcribing a set of orders before you take a break.
4. Follow the 10 steps of transcription, and never sign off on orders before you have ensured that each step has been completed.

🖉 TAKE NOTE

See the HUC job description with implementation of the EMR and CPOE (on p. 9-10 in Chapter 1) for additional management tasks that may be added to the HUC workload with the use of EMR c̄ CPOE.

Time Management

The ability to manage time may be the single most important skill required for successful health unit coordinating.

Time Management Techniques

- Plan for rush periods (e.g., doctors' rounds, afternoons when patients are admitted).

- Plan a daily schedule for the routine tasks.
- Group activities (check charts for new forms when you are transcribing orders).
- Complete one task before you begin another.

The Patient's Chart

Basic Rules That Govern How Notations Are Made in the Paper Chart

- All paper chart form entries must be made in ink. This is done to ensure permanence of the record. Black ink is preferred by many health care facilities because it produces a clearer picture when the record is microfilmed, faxed, or reproduced on a copier.
- Written entries on paper chart forms must be legible and accurate. Diagnostic reports, history and physical examination reports, and surgery reports usually are typewritten or are computer generated.
- Recorded entries on the paper chart may not be obliterated or erased. The method recommended for correcting errors is outlined later in this chapter.
- All written entries on paper chart forms must include the date and time (military or traditional) the entry was made (Fig. 4-1).
- Abbreviations may be used in keeping with the health care facility's list of "approved abbreviations."

Guidelines for Entering Information Into the Electronic Medical Record

- All entries into the EMR/chart must be accurate.
- Handwritten progress notes, electrocardiograms, and outside records and reports must be scanned into the electronic record.
- Errors made in care or treatment must be documented and cannot be falsified.

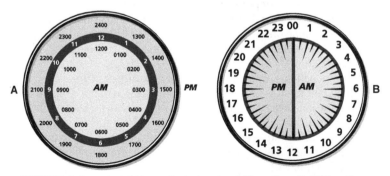

FIGURE 4-1 ▲ **A,** A 24-hour clock showing military time. **B,** Military time.

- All entries into the EMR must include the date and time (military or traditional) of the entry.
- Abbreviations may be used in keeping with the health care facility's list of "approved abbreviations."

Standard Chart Forms

Standard patient chart forms are included in all inpatient paper charts and may vary from one hospital to another. An EMR would include these forms or similar forms accessible by computer.

Forms that are generated by the admitting department include the following:

- Face sheet (also called the information form)
- Conditions of admission form
- Advance directive checklist
- Patients' rights and a notice of the facility's privacy practices (given to patient)

Supplemental Patient Chart Forms

Supplemental patient chart forms are additional to the standard chart forms and are added to patients' charts according to specific care and treatment provided. When the EMR is implemented, information is entered into the patient's EMR or similar electronic forms.

Maintaining the Patient's Paper Chart

As the person in charge of clerical duties on the nursing unit, the HUC is responsible for maintaining the patient's paper chart and performs the following tasks:

- Places all charts in proper sequence (usually according to room number) in the chart rack when they are not in use.
- Places new chart forms in each patient's chart before the immediate need arises.
- Places diagnostic reports in the correct patient's chart behind the correct divider. Matches the patient's name on the report with the patient's name on the front of the chart (the HUC does not depend on room numbers because patients often are transferred to another room).
- Reviews patients' charts frequently for new orders (always checks each chart for new orders before returning them to the chart rack).
- Properly labels the patients' charts so they can be located easily at all times.
- Checks each chart to ensure that all forms are labeled with the correct patient name (chart forms should be arranged in the proper sequence).

- Checks charts frequently for patient information forms or face sheets (usually, five copies are maintained in the chart; doctors may remove copies for billing purposes).
- Assists doctors or other professionals in locating patients' charts.

Splitting, or Thinning, the Paper Chart

The HUC may "thin," or "split," the chart. A doctors' order is not required to thin a patient's chart. In thinning the chart, certain categories of chart forms may be removed and placed in an envelope for safekeeping on the unit.

The following guidelines may be used when a patient's paper chart is thinned:

- Remove early graphic records, nurses' notes, medication forms, and often other forms that are no longer needed in the chart binder. (Check the hospital policy and procedure manual to verify which forms may and may not be removed.)
- Place the removed forms in an envelope.
- Place the patient's ID label on the outside of the envelope.
- Write "Thinned chart" and record the date with your first initial and last name on the outside of the envelope.
- Place a label stating that the chart was thinned, along with the date and your first initial and last name, on the front of the patient's chart.
- If the patient is transferred to another unit, transfer the envelope with the patient chart. When the patient is discharged, return all thinned out forms to the chart in proper sequence.

Summary

The patient's chart (paper or electronic) is a record of care rendered and the patient's response to care during hospitalization. When the EMR is implemented, all health care information is entered or scanned into the patient's chart. The patient's medical information (paper or electronic) constitutes a legal record and should be maintained as such.

CHAPTER 5

Understanding Workplace Behavior, Ethics, and Legal Issues

Workplace Behavior

Factors that influence a person's workplace behavior include the following:
- The organization's philosophy and standards
- The supervisor's leadership style
- How meaningful or important the work is to the person
- How challenging the work is for the person
- How the person gets along with coworkers
- The individual's personal characteristics, such as
  - Ability and aptitude
  - Interests
  - Values
  - Expectations

Health unit coordinators (HUCs) have many job options throughout the health care field. It is important for the HUC to match their particular needs and desires with the appropriate type of position.

How Values Influence Interactions in the Health Care Setting

An individual's values generally are formed by the age of 6 and are influenced by parents, siblings, extended family, friends, peers, and teachers. Significant emotional life events can change values later in life, however.

Life experiences can change what people view as most important, helping them gain empathy for others.

Values have a major impact on how people relate to others, as well as on the choices and decisions that each person makes.

A patient's values can influence the behavior of medical professionals when the values of the two people come into conflict. Value conflicts may arise from cultural, religious, social, or ethnic differences.

Values clarification is an important tool that HUCs can use to prepare themselves to become competent professionals. Examining his values and committing to a virtuous value system will assist the HUC one's in making ethical decisions. It is essential for HUCs to understand and be aware of their values and remain nonjudgmental of others' values that differ from their own.

Workplace Ethics

Workplace ethics are defined as a person's moral values regarding work.

Workplace Ethics for the HUC

- **Dependability**—Patients and members of the health care team rely on the HUC to report to work when scheduled and to be on time. The HUC is also depended upon to perform duties and tasks as assigned and to keep obligations and promises. Getting adequate sleep and staying drug free are essential for the HUC who strives to maintain their dependability. Lack of sleep, use of nonprescription drugs, or misuse of prescription drugs would endanger patients as well.
- **Accountability**—Part of being dependable is being accountable. Accountability means taking responsibility for one's actions and being answerable to someone for something one has done. One must be aware of and must never exceed the scope of practice. If one is unable to report to work or do the job, it is their responsibility to communicate this to the staffing office at least 2 hours before the start of the scheduled shift.
- **Consideration**—Be considerate of the physical and emotional feelings of patients and coworkers.
- **Cheerfulness**—Greet and converse with patients and others in a pleasant manner. Do not bring personal problems to work. Sarcasm, moodiness, and a bad temper are inappropriate in the workplace.
- **Empathy**—Make every attempt to see things from the point of view of patients, families, and coworkers. Keep in mind that stress and worry can affect people's behavior, and refrain from taking a display of anger and frustration as a personal attack.
- **Trustworthiness**—The employer, patients, and coworkers have placed their confidence in the HUC to keep patient information confidential. HUCs are privy to a lot of information and cannot engage in gossip regarding patients, coworkers, doctors, or the hospital.
- **Respectfulness**—Respect, which is a primary value in health care, can manifest in many ways, including tone of voice, body language, attitude toward others, and willingness to work. All life is worthy of respect. We all have a right to our value system and must respect that others have a right to their own. Make every attempt to understand the values and beliefs of patients and coworkers.

- **Courtesy**—Be polite and courteous to patients, families, visitors, coworkers, and supervisors. Address people by name, for example, *Mrs. Johnson* or *Dr. Smith.*
- **Tactfulness**—Be sensitive to the problems and needs of others. Be aware of what is said and how it is said.
- **Conscientiousness**—Be careful, alert, and accurate in following orders and instructions. Never attempt to perform a procedure or task that you have not been trained or, if necessary, licensed to perform.
- **Honesty**—Be sincere, truthful, and genuine, and show a true interest in relationships with patients, families, visitors, and coworkers. If an error is made, bring it to the attention of the appropriate person(s). Never attempt to cover up an error!
- **Cooperation**—Be willing to work with others, especially in the team-oriented climate of health care. When coworkers work as a team, everyone involved benefits.
- **Attitude**—Attitude is a manner of thought or feeling in one's behavior that can be seen by others. Tone of voice and body language can change the message that one is trying to send. One's attitude is reflected in their work. Be positive about your job and the contributions that you are making.

Workplace Appearance

A professional appearance will earn the trust, respect, and confidence of employers, coworkers, patients, and others. A professional appearance also demonstrates self-confidence and sends a message of self-respect and respect for one's position. Follow the dress code outlined in the policy and procedure manual of the facility where you are employed.

General Guidelines for Workplace Appearance

- **Female**—Clothes or uniforms should fit well, should be modest in length and style, and above all should be clean, mended, and wrinkle free. Color and design of undergarments should not be visible through your clothes or uniform. When business dress is called for, slacks or skirts are appropriate with a blouse or sweater. Denim is usually not acceptable.
- **Male**—Slacks and shirt or sweater should fit well, and they should be clean and pressed.
- **Female and Male**—Shoes should be clean and appropriate, as defined in the dress code. Most facilities do not allow open-toe or open-heel shoes. Most nursing personnel wear white tennis shoes (not hightops) for comfort.
- **Female**—Socks/stockings should be worn, especially with a skirt or dress.
- **Male**—Socks should be worn.

- **Female and Male**—Jewelry worn should be modest. Body piercing may or may not be acceptable in your chosen place of employment. Some earrings will interfere with talking on the telephone.
- **Female and Male**—Tattoos may or may not be acceptable in your chosen place of employment.
- **Female and Male**—Hair should be clean and well groomed. Control long hair to keep it out of your face and off of your collar.
- **Female**—Sculptured nails and nail polish are not acceptable for health care workers. Sculptured nails and chipped nail polish provide a place for microorganisms to grow.
- **Female**—Makeup should be modest in amount and color.
- **Female**—Perfume, cologne, and hair spray should be very light or should not be worn at all.
- **Male**—Aftershave, cologne, and hair spray should be very light or should not be worn at all. Patients with respiratory problems, allergies, or nausea could experience ill effects from the aroma.

Cell Phone Use

Everyone has encountered the rudeness of cell phone users who talk loudly while standing in the middle of the walkway at the mall, blocking doorways while talking on the phone, talking loudly in restaurants while others are trying to have a quiet meal, or talking or texting while driving, thereby slowing traffic and not paying attention. Cell phones are heard ringing in hospitals, movie theaters, school classes, and airplanes, and even at funerals. Some often forget about others' personal space, and boundaries.

Cell phones are banned for personal use on hospital units. Ringing cell phones and conversations are annoying and distracting to nursing unit personnel, as well as to patients in nearby rooms.

Cell phones should be turned off while one is working on the nursing unit.

Calls recorded on voice mail may be listened to during breaks. If an important call is expected, phones may be placed on vibrate and taken off of the nursing unit.

Text messaging also is banned while one is working on the nursing unit. Full attention is expected and should be given to your work responsibilities.

Elevator Etiquette

Hospital elevators are very busy places, and it is important to know appropriate elevator etiquette:
- When the elevator button is lit, it is not necessary to continue to push the button; this may be causing the door to close on someone on another floor who is trying to enter or exit the elevator.
- When the elevator does arrive, stand aside and allow people to exit before you try to enter.

- When you are riding on an elevator and are going to a higher floor in the building, stand to the side or in the back so others may exit on their floors.
- Patients who are being transported on stretchers and personnel who are pushing hospital equipment have priority for using elevators.

Health Care Ethics

Ethics is that part of philosophy that deals with judgments about what is right or wrong in given situations. Each health care profession has a code of ethics that has been derived from a set of basic principles that define the concepts of right or wrong for that profession. The National Association of Health Unit Coordinators (NAHUC) has an established code of ethics that can be found in Appendix F.

Ethical Principles for Patient Care

Six basic ethical principles surround the professional care of patients in any health care facility:

1. **Respect**—The patient has the right to considerate and respectful care. Health care workers must provide services with respect for human dignity and the uniqueness of each patient, unrestricted by consideration of the patient's social or economic status or personal attributes, or the nature of the patient's health problem(s).

2. **Autonomy**—The patient is free to choose and implement his own decisions. Part of the patients' bill of rights states that they have the right to refuse treatment to the extent permitted by law and the right to be informed of the medical consequences of their actions. This right does not judge the quality of a decision made by a patient to refuse treatment—it only states that the patient has the right to make the decision. This is the process of autonomy at work. From this basic principle, we have derived the rule involved in informed consent.

3. **Veracity**—The principle of veracity requires that health professionals disclose the truth so the patient can practice autonomy, and that the patient be truthful so that appropriate care can be given. Although health professionals may feel justified in lying to a patient in some situations to avoid some greater harm, other alternatives must be sought.

4. **Beneficence**—Any action that a health care professional takes should benefit the patient. This principle creates a greater ethical dilemma for clinical practitioners than for HUCs. The dilemma arises because of the advanced technology that is available to practitioners today. In cases in which a patient is maintained on life support machines and is in a coma or vegetative state, is it of benefit to maintain the patient on these machines? It is vitally important that patients understand their treatment options, and that they be counseled to speak with loved ones and to complete the appropriate advance directives.

5. **Nonmaleficence**—This principle, which comes from the Hippocratic Oath, means that a health professional will never deliberately inflict harm on the patient. Beneficence, although similar to nonmaleficence, indicates a positive action. The HUC's obligation to nonmaleficence occurs during the act of transcribing orders because an error could result in harm to the patient.
6. **Confidentiality**—Principle 2 of the NAHUC Code of Ethics and the "Patients' Bill of Rights" of the American Heart Association (AHA) outline the individual's right to privacy in health care. HUCs who breach the confidentiality of a patient's medical record have not only violated ethical standards but may well have violated the law.

Patient Care Partnership/Patients' Bill of Rights

Patient expectations and rights include high-quality hospital care, a clean and safe environment, and involvement in care, protection of privacy, help when leaving the hospital, and help with billing claims. The patients' bill of rights has been adopted and modified many times.

In 1998, an Advisory Commission on Consumer Protection and Quality in the Health Care Industry appointed by the President of the United States issued a Patients' Bill of Rights. The Joint Commission (formally the Joint Commission on Healthcare Accreditation) now requires that all hospitals have a bill of rights and a notice of the facility's privacy practices. Copies must be given to each patient or parent of the patient on admission. Additionally, a copy of the bill of rights should be posted at entrances and in other prominent places throughout the hospital. The patients' bill of rights varies in wording among hospitals, but all are based on the following basic ethical principles.

Patients' Bill of Rights

I. Information Disclosure
You have the right to receive accurate and easily understood information about your health plan, health care professionals, and health care facilities. If you speak another language, have a physical or mental disability, or just do not understand something, assistance will be provided so you can make informed health care decisions.

II. Choice of Providers and Plans
You have the right to a choice of health care providers that is sufficient to provide you with access to appropriate high-quality health care.

III. Access to Emergency Services
If you have severe pain, an injury, or a sudden illness that convinces you that your health is in serious jeopardy, you have

(Continued)

Patients' Bill of Rights—Cont'd

the right to receive screening and stabilization emergency services whenever and wherever needed, without prior authorization or financial penalty.

IV. Participation in Treatment Decisions

You have the right to know all your treatment options and to participate in decisions about your care. Parents, guardians, family members, or other individuals that you designate can represent you if you cannot make your own decisions.

V. Respect and Nondiscrimination

You have a right to considerate, respectful, and nondiscriminatory care from your doctors, health plan representatives, and other health care providers.

VI. Confidentiality of Health Information

You have the right to talk in confidence with health care providers and to have your health care information protected. You also have the right to review and copy your own medical record and to request that your physician amend your record if it is not accurate, relevant, or complete.

VII. Complaints and Appeals

You have the right to a fair, fast, and objective review of any complaint you may express against your health plan, doctors, hospitals, or other health care personnel. This includes complaints about waiting times, operating hours, the conduct of health care personnel, and the adequacy of health care facilities.

From the Advisory Commission on Consumer Protection and Quality in the Health Care Industry, 1998. Available at: http://www.consumer.gov/ qualityhealth/rights.htm

Advance Directives

The term *advance directive* refers to an individual's desires regarding end-of-life care and if they should become incapacitated. An adult witness or witnesses or a notary must sign an advance directive. The notary or witness cannot be the person named to make the decisions or the provider of health care. If only one witness is present, it cannot be a relative or someone who will be the beneficiary of property from the patient's estate if the patient dies. Most states require that patients be asked if they have or would like to have an advance directive document.

Advance directives include the following documents:

- A **living will** is a declaration made by the patient to family, medical staff, and all concerned with the patient's care stating what is to be done in the event of a terminal illness. It directs the withholding or withdrawing of life-sustaining procedures. The patient may also define what is meant by *meaningful quality of life*, a phrase commonly used in living wills when the level of functioning that the patient would be comfortable with is described.

- **Power of attorney for health care** allows the patient to appoint another person or persons (called a *proxy* or *agent*) to make health care decisions for the patient should the patient become incapable of making decisions. The proxy (agent) has a duty to act consistently with the patient's wishes. If the proxy does not know the patient's wishes, the proxy has the duty to act in the patient's best interests.

An advance directive becomes effective *only* when the patient can no longer make decisions for himself or herself. The patient may change or destroy any directive or living will at any time.

Health Insurance Portability and Accountability Act (HIPAA) of 1996

The American Health Insurance Portability and Accountability Act of 1996 (HIPAA) is a set of rules to be followed by doctors, hospitals, and other health care providers. The purpose of this law is to protect private individual health information from being disclosed to anyone without the consent of the individual. Except under unusual circumstances, consent must be given in writing. Private information can be used in research studies if it is "de-individualized," so that the identity of the individual cannot be ascertained from the information disclosed.

Under HIPAA, individuals have the right to do the following:

- Obtain notice of the health provider's privacy practices
- Request restrictions on who is allowed to access their health information
- Access, inspect, or copy their personal health information
- Request an accounting of all disclosures of their health information
- Request corrections or amendments to their health information
  Health care providers are required to do the following:
- Provide security for both paper and electronic individual health information
- Institute a complaint process to investigate complaints
- Train staff regarding the law

HIPAA Patient Privacy Rule

This rule was implemented on April 14, 2003.

The HIPAA Patient Privacy Rule establishes regulations for the use and disclosure of *protected health information (PHI)* and mandates that all patients be provided a copy of privacy policies when treated in a doctor's office or when admitted to any health care facility.

When admitted to the hospital, patients will be given a facility directory opt-out form to sign that indicates whether they wish to be listed in the hospital directory. If the patient chooses not to be listed, their chart is labeled *no information/no publication (NINP)*, meaning that no information will be provided to anyone who calls (and it will not be stated whether the patient is in the hospital).

HIPAA Patient Security Rule

This rule is a key part of HIPAA; it became effective as of April 21, 2005.

The HIPAA Patient Security Rule applies to electronic protected health information (EPHI), which is individually identifiable heath information (IIHI) in electronic form. IIHI relates to (1) an individual's past, present, or future physical or mental health or condition, (2) provision of health care to an individual, and (3) past, present, or future payment provided for provision of health care to an individual.

Its primary objective is to protect the **confidentiality**, integrity, and availability of EPHI when it is stored, maintained, or transmitted.

Covered entities (CEs) must comply with the Security Rule. These include health plans (e.g., health maintenance organizations [HMOs], group health plans), health care clearinghouses (e.g., billing and repricing companies), and health care providers (e.g., doctors, dentists, hospitals) who transmit any EPHI.

Confidentiality

The HUC has access to a great deal of PHI and IIHI because of the very nature of the job; this information must be treated with absolute confidentiality by all health personnel. All health care personnel are required to sign a confidentiality agreement upon initiation of employment.

A HUC has two responsibilities in ensuring the confidentiality of patient information: (1) to avoid verbally repeating confidential information, and (2) to control the patient's paper chart or manage the patient's electronic record in a manner that ensures confidentiality of its contents.

Guidelines for Maintaining Patient Confidentiality

- **Do not discuss patient information** (other than what is necessary to care for the patient). All patient information is confidential.
- **Conduct conversations with other health care personnel outside of the hearing distance of patients and visitors**. Do not hold conversations about patient information in the hallways or the cafeteria, or away from the hospital. Be aware of the identity of others who are at the nurses' station during discussions regarding patients.
- **Do not discuss medical treatment with the patient or with relatives** (unless specifically instructed to do so by the doctor or the nurse).
- **Do not discuss general patient information**. Often, hospital personnel, other patients, visitors, or your own friends, relatives, or neighbors may ask you questions regarding a specific patient (especially if the patient is a celebrity) out of curiosity. Politely refuse

to give out the information, and then quickly change the discussion to another subject.

- **Do not discuss hospital incidents away from the nursing unit.** Discussing code arrest procedures, unexpected death, and similar information with persons other than health professionals or within hearing distance of others may instill fear in them regarding health care; such apprehension may even cause them to delay necessary health treatment in the future.
- **Refer to the nurse manager all telephone calls from reporters, police personnel, legal agencies, and other investigative sources.** If in doubt about the authenticity of a telephone caller, obtain information from the caller so you may return the call. After you have had time to confirm the caller's identity, call him back.

Guidelines for Maintaining Confidentiality of the Patient's Paper Chart

- **Follow the hospital policy for duplicating portions of the patient's chart.** Duplication of the patient's chart forms may be the responsibility of the HUC or the health information management department of the hospital. (Read the hospital policy and procedure manual to determine policy regarding copying a patient's chart.)
- **Control access to the patient's chart.** Only authorized persons, such as doctors and hospital personnel, should have access to the chart. Always know the status of the person who is using the chart at the nurses' station. If a patient requests to see his chart, advise the patient that you will notify the nurse and/or doctor. A patient has a legal right to see his own chart, but the doctor may need to write an order, and the doctor or the nurse will go over the information in the chart with the patient.
- **Ask outside agency personnel for picture identification.** It is the responsibility of outside agency personnel to show the HUC picture identification; if they fail to do this, the HUC must ask to see identification.
- **Control transportation of the patient's chart.** Never send the patient's chart to another department through the pneumatic tube system. Do not give patients their charts to hold while they are being transported from one area of the hospital to another.

Managing the Patient's Electronic Record

Access to the patient's EMR may be limited.

The HUC is privy to demographic protected patient information and is responsible for scanning reports, handwritten progress notes, and so forth.

It is the responsibility of the HUC to protect and maintain the patient's confidentiality by being aware of who is in the nursing station looking over their shoulder and/or eavesdropping on conversations.

Tips for Avoiding Legal Problems

■ Know your job description. Do not engage in activities outside your job description.

■ Keep current with the employing agency's policies and procedures. If you believe the policies and procedures are outdated, bring them to the employer's attention, and participate in the revisions.

■ Keep current in your practice. If called upon to do something you are not qualified to do, obtain training. Standard of Care for HUCs may be found in Appendix F. Continued education is a must for all health care workers. Obtain proper training before assuming any position.

■ Do not assume anything. Question orders, policies, and procedures that do not seem appropriate. Do not do something unless you are sure you know how to do it. Ask questions; it is the biggest safeguard.

■ Be aware of relationships with patients. Patients who feel you truly care and have tried to help them to the best of your abilities are less likely to see a lawyer if a problem arises.

In any of the potential problem areas that you may encounter while working as an HUC, apply good judgment, honesty, and reasoning to come up with a moral and ethical way to resolve the conflict.

Summary

The modern health care professional is called upon to exercise professional behavior and judgment in many complex situations. By applying an understanding of confidentiality, legal duty, and ethical responsibility, one will be able to legally and morally fulfill all professional obligations.

CHAPTER 6

Handling Infection Control, Emergencies, and Incident Reports

Infection Control

Patients in all health care facilities are at increased risk of acquiring infection because of their lower resistance to infectious microorganisms, increased exposure to numbers and types of disease-causing microorganisms, and any invasive procedures performed on them. The presence of pathogens in the health care facility does not, however, mean that all, or even most, patients will develop an infection. Development of an infection depends on six components, called the *chain of infection*, as shown in Fig. 6-1.

The six components of the chain of infection include the following:

1. Infectious agent or pathogen (bacteria)
2. Reservoir or source in which the pathogen can live and grow (e.g., human body, contaminated water or food, animals, insects)
3. Means of escape (e.g., blood, urine, feces, wound drainage)
4. Route of transmission (e.g., air, contact, body excretions)
5. Entry way (e.g., mouth, nostrils, breaks in the skin)
6. Susceptible host (individual who does not have adequate resistance to the invading pathogen)

Prevention and control techniques include those listed here:

- Standard precautions
- Airborne precautions
- Good hand washing technique

✐ *TAKE NOTE*

Development of infection can be stopped by breaking the chain of infection. This is accomplished when health care workers follow infection prevention and infection control techniques, thereby preventing the spread of microorganisms to patients and themselves.

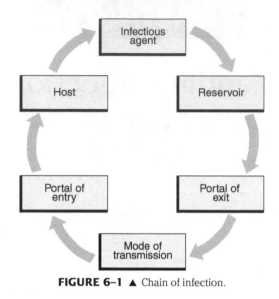

FIGURE 6-1 ▲ Chain of infection.

Records are kept of infectious diseases that occur at a health care facility. The health unit coordinator (HUC) is often responsible for submitting this report to the Infectious Disease department or the infection control officer at the hospital or other health care facility. Most hospitals employ an epidemiologist or infection control officer who maintains all infection records and investigates all hospital-acquired infections. Infection control is essential to providing a safe environment for both patients and health care workers.

Nosocomial Infections

Nosocomial infections are infections acquired from within the health care facility that often are transmitted to the patient by health care workers. Three pathogenic microorganisms that are frequently responsible for hospital-acquired infections are *Streptococcus, Staphylococcus,* and *Pseudomonas.* Excellent hand washing technique is the best way for health care workers to stop the spread of nosocomial infection.

Methicillin-resistant *Staphylococcus aureus* **(MRSA)** is a variation of the common bacterium, *Staphylococcus aureus.* It has evolved the ability to survive treatment with beta-lactam antibiotics, including penicillin and methicillin. In hospitals, patients with open wounds and weakened immune systems are at greater risk for infection than the general public. Hospital staff members who do not follow proper sanitary procedures may inadvertently transfer bacterial colonies from patient to patient.

Hand Washing

Hand hygiene is the most important intervention for preventing infection because the hands of health care workers are the primary source of disease transmission from patient to patient. Most hospitals have a policy that bans artificial fingernails for all health care professionals because they increase infection rates.

Hands should be washed upon arrival at work, before and after personal breaks, and after handling of any patient specimen (even if bagged). Use soap and scrub between the fingers. Rinse each hand thoroughly with running water from the wrists down to the fingertips. Dry with a clean paper towel, and use the towel to turn off the faucet. Microorganisms also can be transmitted when objects are handled in the nursing station. Clean the telephone receiver with an antiseptic wipe upon arrival and periodically throughout the day. Use an antiseptic solution frequently throughout the day. Avoid putting your hands on your face, in your eyes, or in your mouth while you are on the nursing station.

Standard Precautions

Standard precautions involve the creation of a barrier between the practitioner (health care worker) and the patient's body fluids. Standard precautions are used with all patients in health care settings, assuming that all body excretions and secretions are potentially infectious. Body fluids include blood, semen, vaginal secretions, peritoneal fluid, pleural fluid, pericardial fluid, synovial fluid, cerebrospinal fluid, amniotic fluid, urine, feces, sputum, saliva, wound drainage, and vomitus.

The *barrier* in standard precautions is created by wearing personal protective equipment (PPE) that consists of such items as:

- Gloves
- Gown
- Mask
- Goggles or glasses
- Pocket masks with one-way valves
- Moisture-resistant gowns

Every health care employee should practice standard precautions **as required** with every single patient.

Airborne Precautions/Isolation

Airborne precautions (isolation) are used for patients who have infections that can be transmitted through the air, such as tuberculosis. Airborne precautions reduce the risk that droplet nuclei or contaminated dust particles may travel over short distances (less than 3 feet) and land in the nose or mouth of a susceptible person. The patient is placed in a private room with monitored negative air pressure and high-efficiency filtration.

Reverse isolation is used to protect patients with reduced immune system function by reducing their risk of exposure to potentially infectious organisms. Reverse isolation is also known as immunocompromised isolation.

Diseases that can be Transmitted Through Contact with Blood or Other Body Fluids

Acquired Immunodeficiency Syndrome (AIDS)

Acquired immunodeficiency syndrome (AIDS) is caused by human immunodeficiency virus (HIV), also called human T-cell lymphotropic virus type III (HTLV-III), or the AIDS virus. HIV attacks the immune system and reduces the body's ability to defend itself against infection and disease. HIV-positive individuals, whether or not they have full-blown AIDS, become open to opportunistic infections that are not usually threatening to those with a normally functioning immune system. **HIV is transmitted by blood, vaginal fluids, and semen and is not spread through casual contact.**

HIV/AIDS may be spread in the following ways:

- Sexual activity, homosexual or heterosexual (vaginal, anal, or oral), without use of a condom
- Use of a hypodermic needle previously used for injection into an HIV-positive individual
- From an infected mother to an infant during pregnancy or birth
- Through a blood transfusion
- Through the blood of an infected person that enters another person's bloodstream through a cut or open sore
- Through blood that is splashed into the mouth or the eye

Health care workers must use appropriate PPE when it may be possible to come into contact with body fluids from any patient.

Hepatitis B Virus

Hepatitis B virus (HBV) is an inflammation of the liver that is caused by HBV. Similar to AIDS, hepatitis B is spread by body fluids; it is more highly contagious than AIDS. Guidelines provided by the Occupational and Safety Health Administration (OSHA) mandate that employers provide hepatitis B vaccine for all employees who have an occupational exposure risk. The HUC may perform several tasks involving infection control and isolation protocols, which vary from institution to institution. It is necessary in any health care facility for staff members to have a thorough understanding of infection control policies and standard precautions. Accurate information must be given to inquiring visitors. If you are unable to answer a question or are unsure of what to say, ask a nurse to speak with the visitor. All infectious or communicable diseases on the unit must be reported to the infection control officer.

Always wear gloves when handling or transporting specimens, and practice good hand washing technique throughout the working day. Eating and drinking (open cups) should not be done in the nursing station, nor should contact lenses be handled there. Food should not be stored in refrigerators along with specimens.

Emergencies

Chemical Safety

According to OSHA standards, hazardous chemicals must be labeled with a warning, and a material safety data sheet (MSDS) must be kept regarding each hazardous chemical that states what the hazard is; this practice is helpful in any emergency situation.

Chemicals should not be stored above eye level or in unlabeled containers. Appropriate PPE should be worn when chemicals are used. Spill kits that comply with OSHA guidelines must be available at all times.

Fire and Electrical Safety

A code number, such as Code 1000, or a code name, such as Code Red, usually is used when a fire occurs or a fire drill takes place. The HUC may be expected to assist with any necessary patient evacuation and usually helps nursing personnel to close the doors to patient rooms (if the fire is on a different unit). Most hospitals teach the RACE system of fire emergency actions because it is easy to remember:

R	Rescue individuals in danger
A	Alarm (sound the alarm)
C	Confine the fire by closing all doors and windows
E	Extinguish the fire with the nearest suitable fire extinguisher

Classes of Fire

Class A: wood, paper, clothing
Class B: flammable liquids and vapors
Class C: electrical equipment
Class D: combustible or reactive metals

Disaster Procedure

A disaster procedure is a planned procedure that is carried out by hospital personnel when a large number of persons have been injured. The disaster may occur during a flood, a fire, a bombing, or an accident, such as a train derailment or a plane crash. A group of people exposed to hazardous chemicals would also be considered a disaster situation. Every hospital maintains a disaster plan book. Disaster drills are held once or twice a year to keep hospital personnel informed and in practice. Announcement of a code such as "Code 5000" on the hospital public address system activates the disaster procedure.

The HUC usually is designated to handle communication and to call off-duty health care personnel to assist in caring for hospital patients and disaster victims. The role of the HUC may vary from hospital to hospital.

✐ TAKE NOTE

Fire and disaster drills must be taken seriously so that all personnel will be prepared in case a fire or disaster actually happens.

Guidelines for Electrical Safety

- Avoid the use of extension cords.
- Do not overload electrical circuits.
- Inspect cords and plugs for breaks and fraying.
- Unplug equipment when servicing.
- Unplug equipment that has liquid spilled in it.
- Unplug and do not use equipment that is malfunctioning.

Medical Emergencies

Two medical emergencies—i.e., life-threatening situations—that require a calm approach, swift action, and good communication by the HUC (Procedure 6-1) are cardiac arrest and respiratory arrest (commonly called **code arrests**). In a **cardiac arrest**, the patient's heart contractions

---

PROCEDURE 6–1: **Procedure for Performing Tasks Related to Medical Emergencies**

Task	Notes
1. Notify the hospital telephone operator to announce the code.	**1.** *Notification may be made by pressing a special button on the telephone, stating "Code arrest," and giving the location. Be very specific when stating the unit, such as 4A-Apple, 4B-Boy, 4C-Charlie, or 4D-David. Some health care facilities use the expression "Code blue" to designate a cardiac or respiratory arrest.*

PROCEDURE 6–1: **Procedure for Performing Tasks Related to Medical Emergencies—Cont'd**

Task	Notes
2. Direct the code arrest team to the patient's room.	
3. Remove the patient information sheet from the patient's chart, and take or send the chart to the patient's room.	
4. Notify all doctors connected with the patient's case (attending doctor, consultants, and residents).	
5. Notify the patient's family of the situation if requested to do so.	**5.** *If the HUC does communicate with the family, the conversation should be carried on in as controlled a manner as possible, so as not to cause panic. The dialogue might be, "Mr. Whetstone, your brother's condition has changed, and the doctor thought you would like to know. The doctors are with him now. Will you be coming to the hospital?"*
6. Label all laboratory specimens with the patient's ID label, enter the test ordered into the computer, and send the specimen to the laboratory stat.	
7. Call the appropriate department for treatments and supplies as needed.	**7.** *Usually, Cardiopulmonary (Respiratory Care), Diagnostic Imaging, and CSD are the departments involved.*

(Continued)

PROCEDURE 6–1: **Procedure for Performing Tasks Related to Medical Emergencies—Cont'd**

Task	Notes
8. Alert the Admissions department and the ICU about the possibility of transfer to ICU.	**8.** *If the code procedure is successful, the patient is transferred to ICU or possibly CCI to be monitored closely.*
9. For a successful code, follow the procedure for transfer to another unit.	**9.** *See Procedure 9-4 later in this book.*
10. For an unsuccessful code procedure, follow the procedure for postmortem care.	**10.** *See Procedure 9-10 later in this book.*

are absent or grossly insufficient, and no pulse and no blood pressure are detected. In **respiratory arrest**, the patient may cease to breathe, or the respirations become so depressed that the patient does not receive enough oxygen to sustain life. Both conditions require quick action by hospital personnel and the use of emergency equipment. Treatment must be instituted within 3 to 4 minutes because the brain cells deteriorate rapidly from lack of oxygen.

✐ TAKE NOTE

It is helpful when the HUC working on a nearby nursing unit offers assistance to the HUC on the unit where the code is announced.

Incident Reports

Incidents may occur among patients, visitors, or health care facility personnel and students. Events other than accidents that occur within the hospital or on hospital property are reportable.

An incident report form should be written for all incidents that occur to anyone, no matter how insignificant they may seem. Documentation of all incidents is important for identifying hazards and preventing continuing problems, and it is useful when a lawsuit arises from them.

- Names and home addresses of witnesses are required in case the incident becomes a lawsuit and the witnesses are no longer employed at the hospital when the case is brought to court.

- The hospitalist, attending doctor, or resident may be called to examine any patient involved in an incident.
- All incidents involving a patient are reported to the attending doctor.
- A copy of the incident report is sent to the nurse manager, and a copy is sent to Risk Management.
- If the incident involves another department, such as Transport, a copy will be sent to that department's manager.
- The incident report never becomes part of the patient's permanent record.
- Employee hospital incidents must be documented and the employee seen by the employee health nurse or doctor to be eligible for coverage by the state Workers' Compensation Commission. Hospital employees who fail to put into writing something that may appear trivial, such as a finger puncture with a needle, have no evidence to present if an infection follows the injury.
- Risk Management personnel may interview witnesses to a patient incident to be prepared for a lawsuit. Risk Management will also study patient incidents to look for any trends and to prevent future similar incidents.
- A supply of incident reports should always be available on the nursing unit.

Special Services

Flowers

When a health care facility is large enough to have a specific area to which all flowers are delivered, the task of delivering the flowers to patients may be assigned to a hospital volunteer. In hospitals in which the representative from the florist delivers the flowers directly to the unit, the HUC should ascertain that the patient is still on the unit or within the hospital before signing for and accepting the flowers.

Flowers are not allowed on some nursing units, such as intensive care or cardiopulmonary (respiratory care) units, and latex balloons are not allowed in most hospitals (especially on pediatric units). If family members are present, flowers and balloons may be sent home with them.

Mail

Mail is delivered to the nursing unit daily. The mail is checked, and the patient's room and bed numbers are written on each envelope. In the event that the patient has been discharged, you should write "Discharged" in pencil on the envelope and return it to the mailroom.

Summary

It is important for the HUC to know the routines and to be able to perform the tasks related to medical emergencies, fires, and disasters. When emergencies occur, there is no time to look in a book for directions about what should be done.

CHAPTER 7

Managing/Transcribing Doctors' Orders

Doctors' Orders

Patient care orders may be provided in one of three ways:
- Computer physician order entry
- Handwritten orders
- Preprinted on a doctors' order sheet

Computer Physician Order Entry

It is predicted that it will take at least 5 years for the electronic medical record (EMR) to be implemented nationwide. Where computer physician order entry (CPOE) is implemented, the health unit coordinator (HUC) will not be responsible for transcribing the doctors' orders. The HUC responsibilities will include managing and maintaining the electronic record.

Handwritten Doctors' Orders

Occasionally, a doctor will write new orders and will forget to flag the chart. Always check for new orders before returning a chart from the counter into the chart rack.

If new orders are recorded at the top of the doctors' order sheet, check the previous sheet to see if the orders are continued. When orders are recorded near the bottom of the doctors' order sheet, make diagonal lines across the space that is left, so new orders will not be recorded there and continued on the following page. When this happens, it is easy to miss the orders at the bottom of the first page.

Preprinted Doctors' Orders

Preprinted orders are transcribed (after they have been completed and signed by the doctor) by the HUC in the same method as handwritten orders.

Categories of Doctors' Orders

- **Standing orders**—remain in effect to provide a service to the patient routinely until the order is discontinued or changed by the doctor
- **Standing prn orders**—remain in effect to provide a service to the patient as needed until the order is discontinued (either expressly by the doctor or automatically as part of the order) or changed by the doctor
- **One-time or short-series orders**—to be provided on a one-time basis or for a short time; automatically discontinued after completion
- **Stat orders**—given or performed immediately, then automatically discontinued

---

✍ TAKE NOTE

A panel of experienced nurses and HUCs developed 10 steps of transcription to reduce the risk of errors. Variety will always be noted between what is done in different classrooms or hospitals, and even in different nursing units within hospitals. Some of these differences may include the following: symbols may be different or may not be used at all, red ink may be used to note orders or black ink only may be the policy, patient ID cards with imprinter machines may be used in place of labels, and different forms may be used. If the EMR is used, the HUC will not have the responsibility of transcribing doctors' orders.
FLEXIBILITY IS THE KEY!

Transcription of Written or Preprinted Doctors' Orders

Ten Steps of Transcription of Handwritten or Preprinted Doctors' Orders

1. Read the complete set of doctors' orders.
2. Order medications by sending or faxing a copy of the doctors' order sheet to the pharmacy department.
3. Complete all stat orders.
4. Place telephone calls as necessary to complete doctors' orders.
5. Select the patient's name from the census on the computer screen, or collect all necessary forms.
6. Order diagnostic tests, treatments, and supplies.
7. Kardex all the doctors' orders except medication orders. (Kardex may be computerized.)
8. Complete medication orders by writing them on the medication administration record (MAR).
9. Recheck performance of each step for accuracy and thoroughness.
10. Sign off on the completed set of doctors' orders.

Box 7-1 offers tips for avoiding errors when transcribing doctors' orders.

BOX 7-1	Tips for Avoiding Errors when Transcribing Doctors' Orders

- Ask the doctor or nurse for assistance if you are unable to read or understand a doctor's order.
- Use patient information from within the chart to select the computer screen or patient ID label.
- Record the sign-off information on the line directly below the doctor's signature.
- Check the previous page for orders when the orders begin at the top of the page.
- Void space if three or more lines are left at the bottom of the doctors' order sheet.

Symbols

After you have completed each part of the transcription process, place a symbol on the doctors' order sheet to indicate task completion. The symbol should be written in black or red ink, depending on hospital policy, in front of the doctors' order.

Through the use of symbols, a written record reveals the steps completed; this reduces the possibility that a step will be forgotten because of interruptions. Omission can cause delays in treatment that may slow down or be harmful to the patient's recovery.

Symbols vary among hospitals; however, the following list presents symbols that are common in many parts of the country:

- **PC** sent or faxed with time and initials—records that pharmacy copy was sent
- **Ord** and/or computer order number—records that item was ordered
- **K.**—records that order was written or discontinued on Kardex
- **M.**—records that medication order was written on the MAR form
- **Called**, Name of person spoken to, and Time—records completion of a telephone call needed to complete the doctors' order
- **Notified**, Name of person notified, and Time—records that the appropriate health care team member has been notified of a stat order

Signing Off on Doctors' Orders

Signing off with date, time, and full signature is the process used to indicate the completed transcription of a set of doctors' orders.

Avoiding Transcription Errors

The importance of accuracy during the transcription procedure is essential in that errors that may cause serious harm to the patient can be avoided.

Avoiding Transcription Errors

Type of Error	Method of Avoidance
Errors of Omission	Read and understand each word of doctors' orders. If in doubt, check with a patient's nurse or the doctor.
	Use symbols. It is especially important to write the symbol after each step of transcription has been completed.
	When new orders are recorded at the top of the doctors' order sheet, check the previous order sheet to see if these orders are continued from the previous page.
	If the set of orders finishes near the bottom of the doctors' order sheet, cross through the remaining space with diagonal lines. This is done so that newly written orders will begin at the top of the new doctors' order form. When orders are recorded at the bottom of one page and are continued on the next, it is easy to miss transcribing those recorded on the first page.
	Record the sign-off information on the line directly below the doctor's signature to avoid leaving space in which future orders could be written and missed.
	Check for new orders before returning a chart from the counter or elsewhere to the chart rack.
Errors of Interpretation	When in doubt about the correct interpretation of doctors' orders, always check with the registered nurse or the doctor.
Errors in Selection of the Patient's ID Label or Errors in Selection of the Patient's Name on the Computer Screen	Compare the patient's name and the hospital number on the order requisition form or on the computer screen with the same information in the patient's chart. Never select computer labels by the patient's room number only.
	Note: Other staff members frequently use the computer to retrieve information and may change screens while orders are being transcribed. Always double-check the patient information when you are entering orders into the computer.
Errors in Selection of the Patient's Kardex Form	Compare the patient's name and the doctor's name on the Kardex form with the same information in the patient's chart. Never select by using room number alone. If the patient has been transferred, the room number imprinted on chart forms may no longer be correct.
	Note: Many nursing staff members use the Kardex for a quick reference and may flip to another patient's Kardex form while orders are being transcribed. Remove the Kardex form from the

(Continued)

Avoiding Transcription Errors—Cont'd	

Type of Error	**Method of Avoidance**
	holder when you are transcribing orders, and return it to its proper place in the Kardex holder when order transcription has been completed.
Errors in Reading the Doctor's Poor Handwriting	When an order cannot be read because of the doctor's handwriting, refer to the progress record form in the patient's chart. The orders are often recorded on this form also, and use of this information may assist you in interpreting the orders on the physicians' order form. If the order remains unclear, ask the doctor who wrote it or the patient's nurse for clarification. If a doctor has a reputation for poor handwriting, ask to read the orders for clarification before the doctor leaves the nursing unit.

Summary

Until the EMR with CPOE has been implemented, the transcription of doctors' orders is the single most responsible task that an HUC performs. An error may result in harm to a patient or extension of his recovery time. Completing the transcription procedure promptly, accurately, and thoroughly is always best practice in providing quality care for patients.

CHAPTER 8

Recognizing Types of Doctors' Orders

Types of Doctors' Orders

In this chapter, commonly seen doctors' orders are categorized and listed, and information is provided regarding the responsibilities of the health unit coordinator (HUC) and which tests/procedures will usually require a prep and/or a consent form. Abbreviations and terms not explained in this chapter are listed and defined in the appendices. More detailed information may be found in *LaFleur Brooks' Health Unit Coordinating*, 6th edition.

> ✍ **TAKE NOTE**
>
> If electronic medical record (EMR) c̄ computer physician order entry (CPOE) is implemented, the responsibilities of the HUC may be more administrative, and actual ordering may be limited to supplies and equipment.

Patient Activity, Patient Positioning, and Nursing Observation Orders

☑ *Doctors' Orders for Patient Activities*

Patient activity refers to the amount of walking, sitting, and so forth that a patient may do in a given period during their hospital stay. The prescribed activity changes to coincide with the patient's stage of recovery.

Examples of Activity Orders

ABR/CBR   BR c̄ BRP
Dangle   BSC

Up c̄ help	Up in chair
Up in hall	Up as tol
Up ad lib	OOB
Amb	May shower

HUC To Do

Write orders on paper Kardex or enter into computerized Kardex (if EMR c̄ CPOE is not implemented). Order supplies as required.

☑ Doctors' Orders for Patient Positioning

Patient positioning is often determined by the nursing staff; however, the doctor may want the patient to remain in a special body position to maintain body alignment, promote comfort, and facilitate body function.

Examples of Patient Positioning Orders

↑ HOB 30°	↑ Lt arm on two pillows
Fowler's position	Log roll
Mobilize lt leg with 4 sandbags	Turn to unaffected side
Flat in bed or keep HOB ↓	Turn q2h

HUC To Do

Write orders on a paper Kardex or enter into computerized Kardex (if EMR c̄ CPOE is not implemented). Order supplies as required.

☑ Doctors' Orders for Nursing Observation

The doctor may wish to have the nursing staff make periodic observations of the patient's condition; these observations are referred to as signs and symptoms.

Examples of Nursing Observation Orders

VS q4h	BP q shift
Orthostatics q shift	Observe for SOB
Apical rate	Check pedal pulse ® foot q2h
Neuro ✓s q2h	I & O
wt daily	Tympanic membrane temp q4h
CVP q2h	Pulse oximetry q4h
Check CMS fingers rt hand	

HUC To Do

Write orders on a paper Kardex or enter into computerizd Kardex (If EMR c̄ CPOE is not implemented). Order tests as required.

Nursing Treatment Orders

☑ *Doctors' Orders for Intestinal Elimination*

Enemas, rectal tubes, and colostomy irrigations are treatments that are used to remove stool and/or flatus (gas) from the large intestine. A doctor's order is required for the administration of an enema, rectal tube, or irrigation.

Examples of Intestinal Elimination Orders

ORE (oil-retention enema)	SSE (soap suds enema)
TWE (tap water enema)	NS (normal saline) enema
Fleet enema	Rectal tube for gas
Harris flush	Irrigate colostomy

HUC To Do

Write orders on a paper Kardex or enter into computerized Kardex (if EMR c̄ CPOE is not implemented). Order supplies as required.

☑ *Doctors' Orders for Catheterization*

Urinary catheterization is the insertion of a latex-free tube called a *catheter* through the urethral meatus into the bladder for the purpose of removing urine. The doctor may order two types of catheterization procedures: **retention** and **nonretention. Retention** catheters may be referred to as **"Foley"** or **"indwelling"** catheters, and **nonretention** catheters may be referred to as **"intermittent"** or **"straight"** catheters.

Examples of Nonretention Catheterization Orders

May cath q8h prn	Straight cath prn
Cath in 8 hr if unable to void	Cath for residual

Examples of Retention Catheterization Orders

Insert Foley	Indwelling cath to st drain
DC cath this AM	Clamp cath 4 hr then drain

Insert Foley cath for residual; if over 200 mL, leave in
DC cath in A.M.; if unable to void in 6 hr, reinsert

The doctor may order the indwelling catheter to be irrigated on an intermittent or continuous basis to maintain patency (to keep the catheter open). This is called a *closed system.*

Examples of Catheter Irrigation Orders

CBI; use NS @ 50 mL/hr   Irrig Foley c̄ NS
Irrig cath prn patency   Intermittent CBI q4h × 6

HUC To Do

Write orders on a paper Kardex or enter into computerized Kardex (if EMR c̄ CPOE is not implemented). Order supplies as required.

☑️ *Doctors' Orders for Intravenous Therapy*

The purposes of intravenous (IV) therapy are to do the following:
- Administer nutritional support such as total parenteral nutrition (TPN)
- Provide for intermittent or continuous administration of medication
- Transfuse blood or blood products
- Maintain or replace fluids and electrolytes

Box 8-1 gives examples of some commercially prepared intravenous (IV) solutions.

BOX 8–1	**Common Commercially Prepared Intravenous Solutions**

- Sodium chloride 0.45% (NaCl 0.45%, or half-strength NaCl)
- Sodium chloride 0.9% (NaCl 0.9%, or normal saline)
- 5% dextrose in water (5% D/W, or D_5W)
- 10% dextrose in water (10% D/W, or $D_{10}W$)
- 5% dextrose in 0.2% sodium chloride (5% D/0.2% NaCl)
- 5% dextrose in 0.45% sodium chloride (5% D/0.45% NaCl)
- 5% dextrose in 0.9% sodium chloride (5% D/0.9% NaCl)
- Lactated Ringer's solution with 5% dextrose (LR/5%D)
- 5% dextrose in 0.2% normal saline
- 5% dextrose in 0.45% normal saline
- Ionosol T
- Isolyte M
- Lactated Ringer's solution

Peripheral Intravenous Therapy

Peripheral refers to blood flow in the extremities of the body. The cannula is inserted into a vein in the arm, hand, or on rare occasion in the foot (adult). A vein in the scalp or the foot often is used when peripheral

IV therapy is administered to infants. The cannula is short—less than 2 inches long—so that it ends in the extremity. It is not threaded to the larger veins or to the heart as in central venous therapy.

Peripheral IV therapy
- Usually is initiated by the nurse at the bedside
- Usually is started in a vein in the arm by venipuncture
- Is used for short-term IV therapy—a week or less
- Is basic and easiest to initiate
- Is commonly used in hospitals
- Is sometimes given through a vascular access device (VAD)

Central Venous Therapy

When central venous therapy is administered, the catheter is inserted into the jugular or subclavian vein or a large vein in the arm and is threaded to the superior vena cava or the right atrium of the heart. A central venous catheter (CVC) is used and is commonly referred to as a central venous line or a subclavian line.

Types of Central Venous Catheters
Peripherally Inserted Central Catheters (PICCs or PICs)
- Initiated by the doctor or by a nurse certified in the procedure at the bedside and require a consent form
- Inserted into the arm and are advanced until the tip lies in the superior vena cava
- X-rayed to verify placement
- Used when therapy is needed for longer than 7 days
- Used for antibiotic therapy, TPN, chemotherapy, cardiac drugs, or other drugs
- Potentially harmful to peripheral veins
- Sometimes used for blood draws

Percutaneous Central Venous Catheters
- Sometimes referred to as a subclavian line
- Initiated by the doctor at the bedside and require a consent form
- Inserted through the skin directly into the subclavian (most common) or jugular vein and advanced until the tip lies in the superior vena cava or the right atrium of the heart
- X-rayed to verify placement
- Used for short-term therapy—7 days to several weeks
- Used for antibiotic therapy, TPN, or chemotherapy
- Sometimes used for blood draws

Tunneled Catheters
- Initiated by the doctor
- Considered a surgical procedure that requires a consent form
- Inserted through a small incision made near the subclavian vein
- Advanced to the superior vena cava

- Devices called *tunnelers* are used to exit the catheter low in the patient's chest
- Allow the patient to administer their own therapy; the tips can be placed under clothing
- Available in types such as Hickman, Raaf, Groshong, and Broviac
- Inserted for long-term IV therapy—longer than a month
- Used for home care, in long-term care facilities, and for self-administration
- Sometimes used for blood draws (usually require a doctor's order)

Implanted Ports
- Require a surgical procedure that is performed by the doctor in a surgical setting
- Inserted into the subclavian or jugular vein
- (Containers) implanted under the skin in the chest wall
- Followed by a closed incision; the devices cannot be seen but can be identified by a bulge
- Differ from other long-term catheters in that there are no external parts
- Do not require daily care
- Used to administer therapy through a special needle that is inserted into the port
- Types include Port-A-Cath, Med-I-Port, and Infus-A-Port
- Used for long-term and or intermittent treatment; they often are used for chemotherapy administration

HUC To Do

- Send/fax pharmacy copy to the pharmacy.
- Write orders on a paper Kardex or enter into computerized Kardex.
- Order supplies (central line tray and an infusion pump) as required.
- Prepare a consent form (if EMR c̄ CPOE is not implemented).

Heparin Lock—Hep-lock (HL) or Saline Lock
- Venous access device (also called an *intermittent infusion device*) that is placed on a peripheral IV catheter when used intermittently
- Used to maintain an intermittent line when IV fluids are no longer needed but IV entry is still required; commonly used for the administration of medication
- Consists of a plastic needle with an attached injection cap
- Also available as a needleless HL
- Kept patent by heparin or saline flushes ordered by the doctor to be administered at specific intervals (flushes may require a doctor's order)

Often, the HUC is required to order IV solutions at specific intervals; therefore, it is necessary to know the length of time it takes the IV to infuse. An IV of 1000 mL running at 125 mL/hr runs for 8 hours (1000 mL ÷ 125 mL = 8 hours). An IV of 1000 mL running at 100 mL/hr would take 10 hours.

HUC To Do

- Send/fax pharmacy copy to the pharmacy.
- Write the orders on a paper Kardex or enter into computerized Kardex.
- Order supplies/equipment (intravenous [IV] pump) as required (if EMR c̄ CPOE is not implemented).

Transfusion of Blood, Blood Components, and Plasma Substitutes

Administration of Blood and Blood Products

- The patient must sign a specific consent form. A refusal form must be signed if the patient refuses to have a blood transfusion.
- A type and crossmatch is performed to determine the type and compatibility of the blood; this is done before the patient receives blood or certain blood components.
- If blood for type and crossmatch is mislabeled when sent to the lab, it will be thrown away and the patient will have to have the blood drawn again, causing a delay in treatment and discomfort for the patient.
- Normal saline solution generally is used along with administration of blood.
- Blood should be stored only in refrigerators designated for blood storage.
- If blood for two different patients is to be obtained from the blood bank at the same time, two different health care personnel should pick up the blood, or two trips should be made.
- Autologous blood or autotransfusion is use of the patient's own blood for transfusion.
- Donor-directed or donor-specific is the use of blood of relatives or friends for a patient's transfusion.
- Blood may be collected by a device called a cell-saver or autotransfusion system during the patient's surgery, to be transfused back to the patient.

HUC To Do

- Send/fax pharmacy copy to the pharmacy.
- Write orders on a paper Kardex or enter into computerized Kardex (if EMR c̄ CPOE is not implemented).

(Continued)

HUC To Do—Cont'd

- Order supplies (an infusion pump) as required.
- Prepare a consent form.
- Send order/specimen for blood product and type and crossmatch as required (always double-check name on the specimen and name on the order).

Blood and Blood Products Seen in Orders

- Packed cells (red blood cells) (frequently used)
- Plasma
- Platelet concentrate
- Whole blood
- Washed cells
- Fresh frozen plasma (FFP)
- Cryoprecipitates
- Gamma globulins
- Albumin
- Factor VIII

Suction Orders

Wall suction is installed at each patient's bedside. Usually, tubing and suction catheters used with wall suction are stored in the nursing unit supply closet or C-locker. Additional tubing or a specific type and/or size of catheter may have to be ordered for a particular patient.

Suction may be

- Ordered by the doctor to remove fluid or air from body cavities and surgical wounds
- Ordered intermittently or continuously and may be accomplished manually or mechanically
- Set up with some types of suction apparatus during surgery
- Initiated by the nursing staff (e.g., gastric suction)
- Applied in three ways for respiratory tract secretions: through the nose, through the mouth, and through an artificial airway

---

HUC To Do

Write orders on a paper Kardex or enter into computerized Kardex (if EMR c̄ CPOE is not implemented). Order supplies as required.

☑ *Doctors' Orders for Heat and Cold Application*

Heat and cold treatments are ordered for the patient by the doctor. Heat treatment is used to promote comfort, relaxation, and healing; to reduce pain and swelling; and to promote circulation. Cold treatment may be used to relieve pain, reduce inflammation, control hemorrhage, and decrease circulation.

Examples of Heat and Cold Orders

Heat Application	Cold Application
Aquathermia pad	Alcohol sponge
Hot compresses	Ice bag
Sitz bath	Hypothermia machine

HUC To Do

Write orders on a paper Kardex or enter into computerized Kardex (if EMR c̄ CPOE is not implemented). Order supplies as required.

☑ *Doctors' Orders for Comfort, Safety, and Healing*

Nursing staff members select and perform many tasks to promote the comfort, safety, and healing of the patient. However, doctors' orders may relate to these areas also.

A variety of specialty beds are available to reduce the hazards of immobility to the skin and musculoskeletal system. Types of specialty beds that may be used include the following:

- Hill-Rom Air Fluidized
- Kinair III, FluidAir Elite
- Clinitron
- RotoRest

Mattresses used to reduce the hazards of immobility to the skin and to the musculoskeletal system include the following:

- Lotus Water Flotation mattress
- Bio Flote (an alternating air mattress)
- Static Air mattress
- Foam mattress

Examples of Orders for Patient Comfort, Safety, and Healing

Air therapy bed	Egg-crate mattress
Sheepskin on bed	Footboard on bed
Foot cradle to bed	Immobilizer to lt knee 20° flexion
Sandbags to immobilize lt leg	OOB with elastic abd binder
Sling to rt arm when up	Thigh high Ted hose to both legs
Soft wrist restraints for agitation	May shampoo hair
Change surgical dressings bid	Pneumatic hose to lt leg
TCDB q2h	ET nurse referral
	(enterostomal therapist)

Give warm water vaginal irrigation in A.M.
Change surgical dressing and record observations bid.

HUC To Do

- Write orders on a paper Kardex or enter into computerized Kardex (if EMR c̄ CPOE is not implememted).
- Order supplies/equipment as required.
- The patient's height and weight are needed when a bed or Ted hose is ordered.

☑ *Doctors' Orders for Blood Glucose Monitoring*

Blood glucose monitoring is routinely performed by the nursing staff (referred to as point-of-care testing [POCT]). Results of the blood glucose level tests are used to administer or adjust insulin dosage according to the doctors' orders.

Two types of blood glucose monitoring monitors are:
- Accu-Chek Advantage (referred to as Accu-Chek)
- One Touch

HUC To Do

Write orders on a paper Kardex or enter into computerized Kardex (if EMR c̄ CPOE is not implemented).

☑ *Doctors' Orders for Nutritional Care*
Standard Diets

Standard hospital diets consist of a regular diet and diets that vary in consistency or texture (clear liquid; solid) of foods. A standard diet also may be called a regular, house, routine, or full diet. Modifications may be added to these diets (e.g., Reg, 2.5 g Na) as follows:
- Regular diet
- Full liquid diet
- Clear liquid diet
- Mechanical soft diet
- Bland diet
- Diet as tolerated (DAT)

Patient-Requested Diets
Vegetarian Diets (limit or exclude animal foods)

Types of vegetarian diets include the following:
- **Ovolactovegetarian**—includes all plant foods, dairy products, and eggs
- **Lactovegetarian**—includes all plant foods and dairy products

- **Vegan**—includes plant foods only
- **Flexitarian**—includes predominantly plant food, along with nonvegetarian foods such as fish or poultry on occasion

Kosher Diet

A **kosher diet** (adheres to the dietary laws of Judaism) involves the following:
- **Species of animals**—only healthy animals that have split hooves and chew their cud (hogs and pigs do not chew their cud); only fish with scales and fins
- **Manner in which food is processed**—animals properly slaughtered; no mixing of milk and meat
- **Time**—leavened product properly disposed of prior to Passover; no food cooked on the Sabbath
- All fresh fruits and vegetables are kosher.
- Unprocessed grains and cereals are kosher.
- Chicken eggs are kosher.

Therapeutic Diet Orders

Therapeutic diets differ from the regular diet in that the foods served are modified to vary in caloric content, level of one or more nutrients, bulk, or flavor. Therapeutic diets have to be ordered by the doctor.
- **Bland**—mechanically, chemically, physiologically, and sometimes thermally nonirritating to the gastrointestinal (GI) tract
- **BRAT (*B*ananas, *R*ice, *A*pplesauce, and *T*oast)**—a short-term nutritional care treatment for patients with diarrhea, gastroenteritis, and some incidences of food poisoning
- **Soft/low residue**—low-fiber, easily digested foods
- **Low cholesterol**—less than 300 mg/day cholesterol, in keeping with American Heart Association (AHA) guidelines for serum lipid reduction
- **Low sodium**—4-g (no added salt), 2-g, 1-g, or 500-mg sodium diets
- **Low protein**—protein intake may be controlled in Parkinson's disease and in chronic kidney disease
- **High fiber**—addition of fresh uncooked fruits, steamed vegetables, bran, oatmeal, and dried fruits
- **Diabetic (American Diabetic Association [ADA])**—food exchanges recommended by the ADA
- **Calorie restricted**—1200-calorie diet; 1400-calorie diet
- **Renal**—controlled in one or more of the following: protein, sodium, potassium, total fluid, phosphorus
- **Cardiac prudent**—variations of the dietary recommendations of the AHA
- **Low fat**—a diet low in fat, saturated fat, and cholesterol
- **High potassium**—a shortage of potassium in body fluids may cause a potentially fatal condition known as hypokalemia, which typically results from diarrhea, increased diuresis, and vomiting

Other Religious Dietary Restrictions

Islam	Christianity	Hinduism	Church of Jesus Christ of Latter Day Saints (Mormons)	Seventh Day Adventists Church
No pork	Minimal or no alcohol	All meats	No alcohol	No pork
No alcohol	Holy day observances may restrict meat		No tobacco	No shellfish
No caffeine			No caffeine	No alcohol
Ramadan				Vegetarian diet encouraged
Fasting sunrise to sunset for a month				
Ritualized methods of animal slaughter required for meat ingestion				

- **Potassium restricted**—some people with kidney disease are advised to avoid large quantities of dietary potassium.
- **Hypoglycemic**—to normalize blood sugar levels, thereby normalizing stress hormones such as adrenaline and cortisol that are thought to be responsible for the symptoms of mood swings, depression, anxiety, phobias, alcoholism, and drug addiction
- **Low carbohydrate**—restricted carbohydrate consumption, based on research that ties consumption of certain carbohydrates with increased blood insulin levels and overexposure to insulin with metabolic syndrome (the most recognized symptom of which is obesity)

Dysphagia Diets
- **Level I (most restricted): severe dysphagia**—patients just beginning to eat by mouth (unable to safely swallow chewable foods and unable to safely drink thin liquids)
  - Thick homogenous semiliquid textures
  - Decreased fiber
  - No coarse textures, nuts, or raw fruits or vegetables
- **Level II (moderate dysphagia)**—can tolerate minimal easily chewed foods and cannot swallow thin liquids safely
  - Thickened liquids with commercial thickener as needed
  - Very thick juices and milk products
  - Decreased fiber
  - No coarse textures, nuts, or raw fruits or vegetables
- **Level III**—difficulty chewing, manipulating, or swallowing foods (patients beginning to chew)
  - Mechanically soft or edentulous diet
  - No tough skins
  - No nuts or dry, crispy, raw, or stringy foods
  - Meats must be minced or cut into small pieces
  - Liquids as tolerated
- **Level IV (least restricted)**—persons chewing soft textures, swallowing liquids safely
  - Soft textures that do not require grinding, chopping
  - No nuts and no raw, crisp, or deep-fried foods
  - Liquids as tolerated

Postop Diet for Gastric Bypass Procedure
- **Stage 1: clear liquids**—begun with 1 ounce allowed; continued for two to three meals
- **Stage 2: gastric bypass liquids**—begun after clear liquids tolerated; continued for 3 to 4 weeks

- **Stage 3: pureed**—begun after postoperative week 4 (4-ounce meals, 6 to 8 times a day); continued for 1 to 2 weeks
- **Stage 4: soft, solids**—begun after postoperative week 6; continued indefinitely

Gastric bypass liquids include nonfat milk, blenderized soups, 100% fruit juice (diluted ½ water, ½ juice), vegetable juice (e.g., V8, tomato), sugar-free Carnation Instant Breakfast powder mixed with nonfat milk, grits, oatmeal, Cream of Wheat, mashed potatoes (thinned down enough that the food can go through a straw), nonfat sugar-free milkshakes, thinned baby food, and sugar-free drinks (e.g., sodas, tea).

Tube Feeding

Tube feeding, also called *gavage*, is the administration of liquefied nutrients through a tube through the
- Nose into the stomach (nasogastric/nasoenteral)
- Abdominal wall into the stomach (gastrostomy), duodenum (duodenostomy), or jejunum (jejunostomy)

Tube feedings may be given by
- Bolus
- Continuous administration
- Cyclic administration

Types of nasogastric or nasoenteral tubes used for feedings include the following:
- Entron
- Dobbhoff
- Levin

More than 50 medical food products are available for tube feeding, and changes are constantly made as a result of new knowledge. Commercialized prepared formulas include the following:
- Isocal HN
- Deliver 2.0
- Ultracal HN Plus
- Pulmocare
- Jevity
- Boost High Nitrogen
- Boost Plus
- Respalor
- Megnacal

Other Nutritional Care Orders

Force fluids	Limit fluids to 1000 mL per day
NPO	NPO midnight
Sips and chips	Have dietitian see patient
Calorie count	

HUC To Do

- Send/fax pharmacy copies to the pharmacy.
- Write orders on a paper Kardex or enter into computerized Kardex.
- Send tube feeding order to the Nutritional Care department (if EMR c̄ CPOE is not implemented).
- Order required supplies/equipment from central service department (CSD) (feeding pump and supplies).

Medication Orders

Medications are ordered automatically when the EMR c̄ CPOE is implemented. When the doctor enters orders directly into the computer, these orders are sent to the pharmacy. The clinical decision support system (CDSS) alerts the doctor of any patient allergies, drug interactions, or problems with dosage.

A computerized medication cart such as a Pyxis or an Accudose, which requires the user to enter a confidential user ID and password to unlock the cart, is typically used to store and dispense medications on nursing units (Fig. 8-1).

Transcribing medication orders may require the HUC or the nurse to write the orders on a medication administration record (MAR). Printed MARs may be provided by the pharmacy each A.M.; new

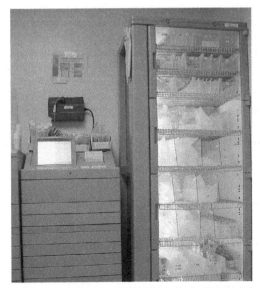

FIGURE 8-1 ▲ Computerized medication cart, including intravenous (IV) solutions.

medications and changes written during the day are transcribed by the registered nurse (RN).

Components of a Medication Order

Each medication order is written with the use of specific components that include directions for the person who is giving the drug. These may be written in slightly different order, but the components remain the same. Box 8-2 provides an example.

BOX 8-2	Five Components of a Medication Order

1	2	3	4	5
Tylenol	325 mg	PO	q4h	WA

The numbered portions of this drug order are as follows:

1. Name of drug	Tylenol
2. Dose of drug (amount)	325 mg
3. Route of administration	PO (by mouth)
4. Time of administration (frequency)	q4h (every 4 hours)
5. Qualifying phrase	WA (while awake)

Naming Medications

Most medications have several names. They are as follows:

1. *Generic name*: A generic drug is the same as a brand name drug in dosage, safety, strength, how it is taken, quality, performance, and intended use. The FDA bases evaluations of substitutability, or therapeutic equivalence, of generic drugs on scientific evaluations. By law, a generic drug product must contain identical amounts of the same active ingredients as the brand name product and must demonstrate the same effect. Generic names are not capitalized.

2. *Chemical name*: The exact designation of the chemical structure of a drug as determined by the rules of accepted systems of chemical nomenclature.

3. *Brand name, trade name, or proprietary name*: The general public often knows the drug best by this name. *The brand name is always capitalized and may have a trademark symbol* (™ *or* ®). Each company that manufactures a drug of the same chemical composition may assign it a brand name. For example, Tylenol, the brand name under which McNeil Laboratories manufactures acetaminophen (its generic name) is named Datril by Bristol Laboratories. *A drug has only one generic name but may have many trade names, depending on how many companies manufacture it.*

   The apothecary system and the metric system are the two methods of weights and measures used in the present-day hospital.

Apothecary System

Measurements in this system are written in lowercase Roman numerals. These numerals have a line over them and may be dotted to avoid confusion with similar-appearing letters or numerals. Also, the unit of measure precedes the numeral. Finally, a medication dosage that is less than 1 is written as a fraction (one-sixth/gram = gr ⅙).

Terms Related to Weight (solid or powder)

Grain (gr)
Dram (dr or ʒ)
Ounce (oz or ℥)

Terms Related to Volume (liquid)

Fluid dram (fl dr or ʒ)
Fluid ounce (fl oz or ℥)
The abbreviation "fl" is not used frequently.

Metric System

The metric system is used everywhere except in the United States. The weight, volume, and measurement units are used in other hospital departments, as well as in the pharmacy. The metric system uses the Arabic numerals—1, 2, 3, and so forth. Abbreviations are placed after the number, as in 50 mg or 500 mL. Quantities less than 1 and fractions are written in decimal form, for example, 0.25 mg, 1.25 mg, and 1.5 g.
- Bicillin 600,000 U bid × 3 days

These basic units are as follows:
- Weight = gram (g)
- Volume = liter (L)
- Length = meter (M)

Smaller and larger units in the metric system can be indicated by attaching prefixes to the basic units. All of the prefixes are not covered because not all are used in doctors' orders.
- To enlarge the basic unit 1000 times, the prefix **kilo-** is added: 1 kilogram (kg) = 1000 g.
- To diminish the basic unit by 100, the prefix **centi-** is added.
- The prefix **milli-** diminishes the basic unit by 1000.
- A milligram (mg), a milliliter (mL), or a millimeter (mm) represents $\frac{1}{1000}$ of the basic unit.
- The symbol "μ" represents the prefix **micro-**. 1 μm = 1 micrometer, or 0.001 millimeter.
- The terms *milliliter (μL)* and *cubic centimeter (cc)* are used interchangeably. 1 L = 1000 cc or 1000 mL.
- *Note*: cc is on The Joint Commission (TJC) "Do not use" list of abbreviations.

Conversion Information

Metric Conversions

Linear Measurements
1 mm = 0.04 in
1 in = 25.4 mm = 2.54 cm
1 m = 39.4 in
1 in = 0.025 m

Volume Measurements
1 tsp = 5 mL
1 tbsp = 15 mL
1 fl oz = 2 tbsp = 30 mL
8 fl oz = 240 mL
1 liter = 1000 mL
1 mL = 1000 microliters
Pint = 473 mL
Quart = 946 mL

Weight Measurements
1 mg = 1000 mcg = 1,000,000
  ng = 0.017 grain
1 grain = 65 mg
1 g = 1000 mg = 0.035 oz
1 oz = 28.3 g
1 kg = 1000 g = 2.2 lb
1 lb = 0.45 kg = 454 g

Percentage Equivalents
0.1% solution = 1 mg/mL
1% solution = 10 mg/mL
10% solution = 100 mg/mL

Routes Most Frequently Used

PO	Orally
Sublingual	Under the tongue
Inhalation	Liquid medications usually administered by the Cardiopulmonary (Respiratory Care) department
Topical	Applied to skin or mucous membrane
Parenteral	By injection or intravenously
Intradermal	Injected between two skin layers
Subcutaneous	Injected under the skin into the fat or connective tissue
Intramuscular	Injected directly into the muscle
IV push	Infused concentrated dose over 1 to 5 minutes
IV piggyback	Intermittent infusion of medication diluted in 50 to 100 mL of solution

Each hospital maintains a schedule of hours for administration of medications. These schedules are set up by the hospital nursing service, and the HUC may be required to learn the hours that are standard for the hospital. Table 8-1 gives examples of time frequencies used to administer

TABLE 8-1	Medication Time Schedule		

Time Symbols	Meaning	Time Schedule	Military Time
qd	Once a day	9:00 AM (anticoagulants: 5:00 PM [daily]—to allow for results of prothrombin time)	0900 1700
		(insulin: 7:30 AM [daily], must be administered before breakfast)	0730
bid	Two times a day during waking hours	9:00 AM and 5:00 PM (9-5)	0900—1700
tid	Three times a day during waking hours	9:00 AM—1:00 PM— 5:00 PM (9-1-5)	0900—1300— 1700
qid	Four times a day during waking hours	9:00 AM—1:00 PM— 5:00 PM—9:00 PM (9-1-5-9)	0900—1300— 1700—2100
ac	½ hour before meals. Varies according to when food cart arrives on unit		
pc	½ hour after meals. Varies according to when food cart arrives on unit		
q3h	Every 3 hours	9:00 AM—12:00 noon–3:00 PM— 6:00 PM—9:00 PM— 12:00 Midnight— 3:00 AM—6:00 AM (9-12-3-6-9-12-3-6)	0900—1200— 1500—1800— 2100—2400— 0300—0600
q4h	Every 4 hours	9:00 AM—1:00 PM— 5:00 PM—9:00 PM— 1:00 AM—5:00 AM (9-1-5-9-1-5)	0900—1300— 1700—2100— 0100—0500
q6h	Every 6 hours	9:00 AM—3:00 PM— 9:00 PM—3:00 AM (9-3-9-3)	0900—1500— 2100—0300
q8h	Every 8 hours	9:00 AM—5:00 PM— 1:00 AM (9-5-1)	0900—1700— 0100
q12h	Every 12 hours	9:00 AM—9:00 PM (9-9)	0900—2100

medications. Remember that this varies among hospitals. Also, military time may be used in place of standard time.

Some qualifying phrases commonly seen include the following:

- For severe pain
- For stomach spasms
- For N/V
- While awake
- For sleep

Refer to Appendix D for a list of commonly ordered medications (brand and generic names) and their uses. More detailed information regarding groups of medications may be found in Chapter 13 of *LaFleur Brooks' Health Unit Coordinating*, 6th edition.

Look- or Sound-Alike Medications

Many drug names look or sound alike. Name confusion is to blame for 12% to 25% of errors voluntarily registered in the United States by health care professionals and patients. Confusion surrounds generic and brand names for medications. The risk is increased when doctors who are writing prescriptions have illegible handwriting. Below are some examples of similarly spelled medications.

Medication Order Written by Doctor	Medication That Could Cause Confusion
quinine 200 mg PO	quinidine 200 mg PO
lamotrigine 150 mg	lamivudine 150 mg PO
Zyrtec 20 mg q day	Zantac 200 mg q day
indapamide 2.5 mg PO	isradipine 2.5 mg PO
Lamictal 25 mg q day	Lamisil 250 mg q day
hydroxyzine 25 mg PO	hydralazine 25 mg PO
Losec TM 20 mg PO qd	Lasix TM 20 mg PO qd
Klonopin 0.5 mg PO	clonidine 0.5 mg PO
Lovastatin 40 mg q day	lisinopril 40 mg q day
Platinol	Paraplatin

"Do Not Use" Abbreviation List, per Requirements of the Joint Commission (TJC)

(Individual health care facilities may have additional unacceptable abbreviations.)

Unacceptable Abbreviations	Acceptable Abbreviations
1.0 mg	1 mg
Zero after decimal	*Do not use terminal zero for dose expressed in whole numbers.*

"Do Not Use" Abbreviation List, per Requirements of The Joint Commission (TJC)—Cont'd

.5 mg *No zero before decimal*	0.5 mg *Always use zero before decimal when the dose is less than a whole unit.*
U or u	Write "unit."
IU (for international unit)	Write "international unit."
μg	Write "mcg" or "microgram."
cc	Write "mL" or "ml," or write "cubic" centimeter or "milliliters."
q.o.d. or QOD *Latin abbreviation for every other day*	Write "every other day."
Q.D. or QD *Latin abbreviation for every day*	Write "daily," "every day," "Q day," or "Q 24 hour."
HS	Write "half-strength."
AU, AS, or AD *Latin abbreviation for both ears, left ear, or right ear*	Write "both ears," "left ear," or "right ear."
TIW	Write "three times a week," or specify days (e.g., Q M-W-F).
MS, MS04, MgSO4	Write "morphine sulfate" or "magnesium sulfate."

The Five Rights of Medication Administration

It is vital that the HUC is accurate when reading and transcribing medication orders. Use the five rights listed below as a guide when transcribing medications.

1. **Right Drug**: Pay close attention to the drug order when transcribing medications. Many drugs have similar names and spellings.
2. **Right Dose**: Once again, accuracy in transcribing the medication dose is vital to patient safety.
3. **Right Time**: Pay special attention to stat or one-time orders, and let the nurse know if a stat or now medication is ordered.
4. **Right Route**: Never assume the route for a medication; always check if the order is not clear.
5. **Right Patient**: Transcribe medication on the correct patient's chart or MAR. Always double-check the name in the chart when transcribing medication orders. If you make an error, correct it immediately and notify the nurse.

Controlled Substances

In 1971, the Controlled Substances Act updated previous laws that regulated the manufacture, sale, and dispensing of narcotics and drugs having potential for abuse. These drugs are referred to as *controlled drugs* or *controlled substances*. Controlled substances are divided into five classes, or schedules. Each of these classes differs according to its potential for abuse; therefore, each is controlled to a different degree. The U.S. Attorney General has the authority to reschedule the class in which a drug is placed, remove a substance from the controlled list, or assign an unscheduled drug to a controlled category. Therefore, the drugs in particular classes are subject to change.

Schedule I

High potential for abuse; usually nonexistent in a health care setting except for specific, approved research. Examples are heroin, marijuana, lysergic acid diethylamide (LSD), peyote, mescaline, psilocybin, methaqualone, and dihydromorphine.

Schedule II

High potential for abuse; may lead to severe physical or psychological dependence. A written prescription signed by the physician is required for Schedule II drugs. In an emergency situation, oral prescriptions for limited quantities may be filled; however, the physician must provide a signed prescription within 72 hours. Prescriptions cannot be refilled. Examples include morphine, codeine, hydromorphone, methadone, meperidine, cocaine, oxycodone, fentanyl, etorphine hydrochloride, anileridine, and oxymorphone. Also included in Schedule II are amphetamines, methamphetamines, phenmetrazine, methylphenidate, glutethimide, amobarbital, pentobarbital, secobarbital, and phencyclidine.

Schedule III

Less abuse potential than those in Schedules I and II. Includes compounds that contain limited quantities of certain narcotic drugs and non-narcotic drugs such as derivatives of barbituric acid (except those in another schedule), methyprylon, nalorphine, benzphetamine, chlorphentermine, clortermine, phendimetrazine, anabolic steroids, paregoric, and any suppository dosage form containing amobarbital, secobarbital, or pentobarbital.

Schedule IV

Less abuse potential than those in Schedule III. Includes barbital, phenobarbital, mephobarbital, chloral hydrate, ethchlorvynol, ethinamate, meprobamate, paraldehyde, methohexital, fenfluramine, diethylpropion, phentermine, chlordiazepoxide,

Controlled Substances—Cont'd

diazepam, oxazepam, clorazepate, flurazepam, clonazepam, prazepam, lorazepam, alprazolam, halazepam, triazolam, mebutamate, dextropropoxyphene, and pentazocine.

Schedule V

Less abuse potential than those in Schedule IV. Consists of preparations that contain limited quantities of certain narcotic drugs, generally for antitussive and antidiarrheal purposes.

Administration of Medications

- As dispensers of controlled substances for medicinal purposes, hospital pharmacies are required to be registered with the Drug Enforcement Administration, which mandates that records be maintained on certain drugs.
- Controlled drugs must be kept in a double-locked cupboard, a medication cart, or a computerized medication dispensing system on the nursing unit.
- If the medications are kept in a computerized medication system, an ID number and password and/or fingerprint identification may be required to access the medication drawers.
- Each time a medication from the locked cupboard or cart is given, the nurse who administers the medication is responsible for writing the required information on the disposition sheet.
- Each drug and each dosage of the drug requires the use of a separate disposition sheet. When the disposition sheet is completed, it is returned to the pharmacy.
- If a computerized system is used, the nurse must verify the count of the medications left in the drawer after removal of the drug.
- The count then is maintained on a computerized log.
- Medications that fall into the category of controlled drugs have an automatic stop date. An automatic stop date means that after a certain period, for example, 72 hours, the drug may no longer be given to the patient unless renewed by a written order.
- Controlled substances usually have a 72-hour limit. Each health care facility develops its own list of drugs that have automatic stop dates. Although other types of drugs are included under the heading "Controlled Substances," narcotics and hypnotics are the most frequently used.

Renewing Medication Orders

Drugs such as narcotics, hypnotics, and other drugs controlled by federal or state laws have an automatic stop date. Hospital medical committees also may set automatic stop dates on anticoagulants and antibiotics.

These drugs must be reordered before or when the stop date is reached. If the doctor wishes to discontinue the medication that is to be renewed, this may be indicated by writing "No" on the renewal stamp or by not signing the renewal stamp. This automatically discontinues the medication.

Discontinuing Medication Orders

If the doctor wishes to discontinue the medication that is to be renewed, "No" may be written or chosen, along with a check mark on the renewal stamp.

When a doctor discontinues a standing or standing prn order, a discontinue order is written on the doctor's order sheet: DC Achromycin 500 mg PO tid.

To discontinue medications on the MAR, indicate "DC" on the correct day and time, and draw a line through the days the medication will not be given. A yellow or pink highlight is usually drawn over the medication entry that is discontinued.

Medication Order Changes

A patient's medication order may have to be changed for any number of reasons.

- The change may involve the dosage, route of administration, or frequency of a drug already ordered.
- Whenever this is done, this is considered a new order and should be written as such on the MAR.
- It is illegal to erase or cross out parts of an order or to write over an order on the MAR, because this is a record of what medication has been administered to the patient. This may result in a serious medication error.
- The old order must be discontinued according to the policy and the new order written.

Total Parenteral Nutrition (TPN) or Intravenous Hyperalimentation

- TPN is the process of intravenously infusing carbohydrates, proteins, fats, water, electrolytes, vitamins, and minerals.
- Nutrients are infused through a catheter that is placed directly into a large central vein and is then advanced into the superior vena cava. The veins most commonly used are the jugular and subclavian veins.
- Usually a long-term therapy, TPN is administered through central venous catheters that are designed for long-term use.
- Requires a written doctors' order (preprinted with numbers filled in by the doctor) and is prepared by the pharmacist under sterile conditions. The solution is kept refrigerated until 30 to 40 minutes before infusion.

- Expensive and time comsuming to make, so it is very important to send new and changed orders immediately to the pharmacy.
- Patients receiving TPN require frequent (daily) blood tests for electrolyte and lipid levels.

HUC To Do

- Send/fax the doctors' orders to the pharmacy.
- Write medications on the MAR (if EMR c̄ CPOE has not been implemented).

Laboratory Orders

Tests performed by the laboratory are ordered for diagnostic purposes and for the evaluation of a prescribed treatment. It is necessary for the HUC to be able to interpret terms the doctor may use to write laboratory orders. For instance,

- **Routine or today**—Usually performed within a 4-hour period
- **Daily**—The test is ordered once by the doctor but is requisitioned each day or entered into the computer for multiple days in advance until the order is discontinued.
- **Stat**—Done immediately; the HUC may need to notify the laboratory by phone or verbally notify the appropriate nursing personnel on the unit.

Specimens

All laboratory tests require a specimen. Specimens usually collected by the nurse include the following:

- Blood (the most common)
- Urine
- Sputum
- Stool
- Sweat
- Wound drainage
- Discharge from body openings
- Gastric washings (lavage)

The doctor usually collects specimens by invasive procedures that enter parts of the body or a body cavity. These are called nonretrievable specimens because they are difficult to replace. Box 8-3 lists considerations for sending specimens to the laboratory.

BOX 8-3 | Sending Specimens to the Laboratory

It is often the HUC's responsibility to take the specimen to the laboratory. This should be done as soon as possible. The pneumatic tube system may be used, but specimens collected by an invasive

(Continued)

BOX 8–3	Sending Specimens to the Laboratory—Cont'd

procedure, such as cerebrospinal and amniotic fluids, should not be sent via the pneumatic tube. When blood or urine specimens are sent by the pneumatic tube system, they must be well wrapped and cushioned.

Types of specimens and the names of procedures used to obtain them

Specimen	Procedure Performed to Obtain Specimen	Required
Spinal fluid	Lumbar puncture; also called *spinal tap*	Consent and tray
Bone marrow	Sternal puncture; also called *bone marrow biopsy*	Consent and tray
Abdominal fluid	Abdominal paracentesis	Consent and tray
Pleural fluid	Thoracentesis	Consent and tray
Amniotic fluid	Amniocentesis	Consent and tray
Biopsy specimen	Biopsy of a part of the body	Consent and tray
Cervical smear	Pelvic examination	Tray

HUC To Do

- Ensure that the specimen is labeled correctly by the nurse or the doctor (should include the date and time collected along with the initials of the person who collected the specimen).
- Ensure that the specimen is bagged.
- Wear gloves when handling specimens (even when nurse or doctor has placed in bag).
- Wash hands after handling specimens (even when nurse or doctor has placed in bag).
- Enter orders into the computer.
- Follow appropriate protocol for specimen handling and sending to the laboratory.

Point-of-Care Testing

Many laboratory tests that were once drawn and analyzed only in the laboratory now may be performed on the nursing unit. A laboratory test that is collected and analyzed on the hospital unit by nursing personnel is called a point-of-care laboratory test. Because point-of-care testing may be ordered, the procedure for ordering a test may change.

Results are obtained through several methods. These include analysis by portable automated analyzers, the use of reagents (chemicals), and microscopic visualization. Portable automated analyzers may be used in departments that require immediate results; they decrease the need for stat specimens to be sent to the laboratory. Some common analyzers are Accu-Chek for blood glucose and i-STAT for activated partial thromboplastin time (APTT) (partial thromboplastin time [PTT]); the analyzer name may be used in the physician's order.

Some tests that may be done on the unit by this method include the following:

- ACT (activated clotting time)
- APTT (PTT)
- Electrolytes
- Blood glucose (sugar)
- BUN (blood urea nitrogen)
- H&H (hemoglobin and hematocrit)
- Human chorionic gonadotropin (hCG)
- Blood and urine monitoring for the presence of ketones and the levels of glucose (i.e., Accu-Chek)
- Stool for guaiac, Gastroccult, or Hemoccult
- Fern test (uses both a reagent and microscopic visualization) to indicate the presence of amniotic fluid
- *Helicobacter pylori* (*Campylobacter*-like organism [CLO] test)—The CLO test actually uses a biopsy specimen obtained in the Endoscopy department and may yield positive results within 2 hours.
- ABGs (arterial blood gases, a pulmonary function test) also may be run on an automated analyzer in the unit

HUC To Do

- Notify the nursing staff if the test is stat.
- Write the orders on a paper Kardex or enter into computerized Kardex (if EMR c̄ CPOE is not implemented).
- Order laboratory test as required (if EMR c̄ CPOE is not implemented).

Divisions Within the Laboratory

(Fig. 8-2)

Hematology

The Hematology division performs tests related to the physical properties of blood (including blood cells and their appearance), tests related to clotting and bleeding disorders, and coagulation (clotting) studies to monitor patients on anticoagulant therapy.

Most of these tests are done on a blood specimen. However, bone marrow and spinal fluid also may be studied in the Hematology division.

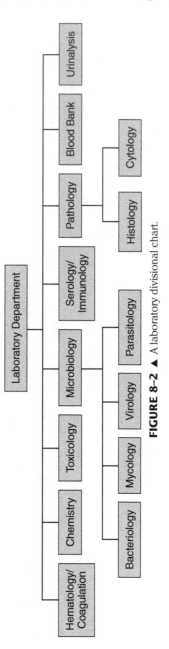

FIGURE 8-2 ▲ A laboratory divisional chart.

(Fasting generally is not required for tests performed in the Hematology division of the laboratory.)

☑ Doctors' Orders for Hematology Studies

It is impossible to list all doctors' orders that relate to this division of the laboratory, so listed here are the more common ones in their abbreviated forms, along with an interpretation for reference purposes:

- PT (prothrombin time)—International Normalized Ratio (INR) may be included
- APTT (activated partial thromboplastin time)
- PTT (partial thromboplastin time)
- Bleeding time or template bleeding time (TBT)
- Clotting time
- CBC (complete blood cell count) or hemogram includes the following tests, which also may be ordered separately (the number of tests included in a CBC may vary among hospitals):
  - Red blood cell count (RBC)
  - Hemoglobin (Hgb)
  - Hematocrit (Hct); also called packed cell volume (PCV)
  - RBC indices
  - White blood cell count (WBC) and Differential (Diff)
  - Blood smear
  - May include platelet count
  - H&H (hemoglobin and hematocrit)
- RBC indices; these include the following:
  - MCH (mean corpuscular hemoglobin—content of hemoglobin in average individual red blood cell)
  - MCHC (mean corpuscular hemoglobin concentration—average per 100 mL of packed red blood cells)
  - MCV (mean corpuscular volume—average volume of individual red blood cells)
  - RDW (red blood cell distribution width)
  - WBC (white blood cell count)
- Diff (differential)—includes various types of WBCs such as the following:
  - Lymphocytes (lymphs)
  - Monocytes (monos)
  - Neutrophils (neutros or segmented neutrophils)
  - Eosinophils (eos)
  - Basophils (basos)
  - Blood smear
  - Platelet count or platelets
  - ESR (erythrocyte sedimentation rate or sed rate); methods such as Westergren or Wintrobe may be specified
  - Retics (reticulocytes or immature red blood cells)
  - LE cell prep (lupus erythematosus cell prep)

HUC To Do

- Notify the clinical laboratory if the test is stat (may require telephone communication).
- Write the orders on a paper Kardex or enter into computerized Kardex (if EMR c̄ CPOE is not implemented).
- Order laboratory test as required (if EMR c̄ CPOE is not implemented).

Chemistry

The Chemistry division performs tests related to the study of chemical reactions that occur in living organisms. When a disease process occurs, chemicals within the body fluids vary from normal. Any variance permits diagnosis or evaluation of the patient's health status.

Whole blood, plasma, or serum, and urine are the specimens most commonly collected for study in this division of the laboratory. Specimens for urine chemistries may require a 24-hour urine specimen. Some specimens that are to be kept for a prolonged period have a preservative added to the collection bottle before it is sent to the unit. Other 24-hour specimens may have to be iced in the patient's bathroom until the collection process is completed. Many blood chemistry tests require the patient to fast or be NPO (nothing by mouth).

☑ *Doctors' Orders for Blood Chemistry Studies*

Frequently ordered blood chemistry tests are listed below, written in abbreviated form as the doctor would write them on the doctors' order sheet. The full name of each test is given in parentheses. Normal values for common blood chemistry studies are given in Box 8-4.

BOX 8-4	Normal Values for Frequently Performed Hematology-Coagulation Studies and Blood Chemistry Studies

Hematocrit (Hct)
Male: 45 to 50 vol/dL
Female: 40 to 45 vol/dL

Hemoglobin (Hgb)
Male: 14.5 to 16 g/dL
Female: 13 to 15.5 g/dL
White blood cell count (WBC): 6000 to 9000 mm^3
Prothrombin time (PT): 12 to 15 sec
Sodium (Na): 132 to 142 mEq/L
Potassium (K): 3.5 to 5 mEq/L
Fasting blood sugar (FBS): 70 to 120 mg/dL

✐ TAKE NOTE

Unless otherwise indicated, the specimen used for the following tests is serum (blood), which is collected by nursing or laboratory personnel.

- Acid phos (acid phosphatase)
- Alk phos (alkaline phosphatase)
- Amylase (serum)
- ALT (alanine aminotransaminase [SGPT])
- AST (aspartate aminotransferase [SGOT])
- Bilirubin (total, direct, or indirect)
- BMP (basic metabolic panel)—Tests may be ordered separately and may include the following:
  - Na (sodium)
  - K (potassium)
  - Cl (chloride)
  - CO_2 (carbon dioxide—dissolved)
  - Glucose
  - BUN (blood urea nitrogen)
  - Creatinine
  - Ca (calcium)
  - BNP (brain natriuretic peptide)
  - BS (blood sugar) or glucose
  Cardiac enzymes (a custom chemistry panel) may involve "isoenzymes" and may include the following tests:
- Creatine phosphokinase (CPK, CK) and CK-MB
- Troponin I or T
- Myoglobin or homocysteine
- Lactate dehydrogenase (LDH)
- Cholesterol (fasting recommended)
- CMP—A comprehensive metabolic panel consists of 14 chemistry tests, including Na, K, Cl, CO_2, glucose, BUN, creatine, Ca, albumin, total bilirubin, alk phos, total protein, AST, and ALT.
- CPK or CK (creatine phosphokinase or creatine kinase)
- Creatinine clearance test—A creatinine clearance test is done to study kidney function. It requires testing of the blood and a 24-hour urine specimen.
  Electrophoresis may include the following:
- Protein electrophoresis
- Lipoprotein electrophoresis
- Immunoelectrophoresis
- FBS (fasting blood sugar) (fasting for 8 to 10 hours is required)
- GTT (glucose tolerance test) (fasting for 8 to 10 hours is required)— The test may be performed over several hours, usually 3 to 6 hours. The patient has an FBS drawn to establish baseline data and then is

given a large amount of glucose solution to drink. Timed blood and urine specimens are taken and labeled by the nurse.

- HbA$_{1c}$, GHb, or GHB (glycosylated hemoglobin)
- HDL (high-density lipoprotein)
  - Isoenzymes (also called *isozymes*)—Isoenzymes or isozymes determine the source (body part enzymes) responsible for the elevation of enzymes such as LDH, CPK, or CK by revealing the variations in these enzymes through tests such as CK-MB.
- LDH (lactate dehydrogenase)
- Lipid panel (fasting recommended)—includes cholesterol, triglycerides, HDL (high-density lipoprotein), and LDL (low-density lipoprotein)
  Lytes (electrolytes) may be performed separately and include the following:
- Sodium (Na)
- Potassium (K)
- Chloride (Cl)
- Carbon dioxide (CO_2)
- PAP (prostatic acid phosphatase)
- PSA (prostate-specific antigen)
- Serum creatinine
- SGOT (serum glutamic-oxaloacetic transaminase); also called aspartate aminotransferase (AST)
- SGPT (serum glutamic-pyruvic transaminase); also called alanine aminotransferase (ALT)
- TIBC (total iron-binding capacity) (fasting recommended)
- Troponin (cardiac test for acute myocardial infarction [AMI])
- 2 hr PP BS (2 hours postprandial blood sugar)—It is the responsibility of the HUC to notify the laboratory when the patient has finished eating. Blood for this test may be drawn 2 hours after any meal and, if ordered for the laboratory to draw, is ordered T/Stat (timed stat) at the specified time.
- Triglycerides (fasting recommended)
- Uric acid

HUC To Do

- Notify the clinical laboratory if the test is stat (may require telephone communication).
- Write the orders on a paper Kardex or enter into computerized Kardex (if EMR c̄ CPOE is not implemented).
- Order laboratory test as required (if EMR c̄ CPOE is not implemented).

Special Chemistry Studies

Many of the tests previously included in the Nuclear Chemistry division of the clinical laboratory or the nuclear medicine laboratory may now be performed through a non-radioisotope–based method and may be included in the Chemistry division as a special chemistry study. These tests usually are listed under the general heading of Chemistry on the computer order screen or on requisitions. The following studies are examples of tests that may be performed by these divisions:

- ACTH (adrenocorticotropic hormone)
- Cortisol
- Folate
- FSH-urine (follicle-stimulating hormone)
- LH (luteinizing hormone)
- Schilling's test
- TBG (thyroxine-binding globulin)
- TSH (thyroid-simulating hormone)
- T_3 (triiodothyronine)
- T_4 (thyroxine)
- T_7 (free thyroxine index)

☑ Doctors' Orders for Urine Chemistry Studies

Urine chemistry tests are listed below:
- Urine glucose
- Urine creatinine
- Urine protein
- Urine osmolality

HUC To Do

- Notify the clinical laboratory if the test is stat (may require telephone communication).
- Write the orders on a paper Kardex or enter into computerized Kardex (if EMR c̄ CPOE is not implemented).
- Order laboratory test as required (if EMR c̄ CPOE is not implemented).
- A paper requisition may be required to accompany the labeled specimen.

Toxicology

Toxicology is the scientific study of poisons, their detection, their effects, and methods of treatment for conditions they produce. Tests for detecting drug abuse and for monitoring drug usage are also performed in toxicology. Special consents, handling, and labeling may be required. Specimens include blood and urine.

☑ Doctors' Orders for Toxicology Studies

To check the maximum and minimum blood levels of certain medications the patient is receiving, the doctor will order peak-and-trough levels.

Trough levels usually require that blood be drawn 15 minutes before the next dose of medication is given to the patient. For peak levels, the blood is usually collected 15 minutes after IV infusion and 30 to 60 minutes after intramuscular (IM) injection. Peak-and-trough levels would be ordered "timed," meaning that the blood should be drawn at the specified time. Random levels (not timed) also may be drawn for toxicology studies.

Examples of Medications Commonly Tested in Toxicology

Antibiotics—Amikacin, gentamicin, kanamycin, and tobramycin are examples of types of medication ordered for peak-and-trough levels.
Anticonvulsants—Dilantin (random)
Cardiovascular—digoxin (random)
Immunosuppressants—tacrolimus (Prograf) (trough level)
Drug screen
ETOH (ethanol or alcohol)

HUC To Do

- Notify the clinical laboratory if the test is stat (may require telephone communication).
- Write the orders on a paper Kardex or enter into computerized Kardex (if EMR c̄ CPOE is not implemented).
- Order laboratory test(s) as required (if EMR c̄ CPOE is not implemented).
- Coordinate the draw time(s) as required for timed specimen(s).

Microbiology

The terms *microbiology* and *bacteriology* sometimes are used interchangeably. However, large laboratories may use the broader term *microbiology* as a division name within the hospital, with areas in that division designated for bacteriology, parasitology, mycology, and virology, to name a few.

Microbiology is the study of microorganisms that cause disease. Specimens are cultured, grown in a reproducing medium, identified with the use of biochemical tests, and then tested for antibiotic sensitivity. Parasites, organisms that live off other living organisms, are dealt with in parasitology. Fecal specimens are studied here for ova and parasites. In **mycology**, cultures are set up to isolate and identify fungi. Because the fungi must grow to produce spores, these cultures may take several weeks. **Virology** is the study of viruses that cause disease. Identification of the exact virus or bacterium that is the causative organism of a specific disease is important in that isolation procedures are based on the methods by which organisms are spread.

Almost any type of specimen may be studied in the Microbiology division, including blood; urine; sputum; stool (feces); catheter tips; and eye, ear, nose, throat, and wound drainage. For microbiology tests, the exact specimen must be included on the requisition. (Fasting is not required for tests performed in the Microbiology division of the laboratory.)

☑️ Doctors' Orders for Microbiology Studies

Frequently ordered tests performed in the Microbiology division are listed below.

Bacteriology

- C&S (Culture and sensitivity)—A C&S can be ordered on any specimen and should be included on the requisition. The specimen is cultured and if organisms grow, they are tested for antibiotic sensitivity; this reveals those antibiotics that should be effective for treatment.
- Cultures (e.g., anaerobic, *Nocardia, Clostridium difficile* [C diff], *Acinetobacter*)
- AFB (acid-fast bacilli) culture (to determine the presence of such acid-fast bacilli as Mycobacterium tuberculosis [TB])
- CC (urine for colony count)
- Gram stain (performed to classify bacteria as Gram-negative or Gram-positive)
- Blood cultures (specimens may be collected as multiple specimens [different times or different sites]) in order to ensure accurate isolation and identification of the causative organism

Parasitology

- Stool for O&P (ova and parasites)—Stool for O&P is usually ordered times three; it requires three different stool specimens (three requisition forms must be prepared) to detect the presence of ova (eggs) or parasites in the stool.

Mycology

- Fungal culture or mycology culture—Results may take several weeks to obtain and may reveal the presence of fungi such as *Histoplasma, Coccidioides,* and *Candida.*

Virology

Virus culture (may be ordered with virus serology)—Virus cultures may be done on any specimen. For serology, see the next section.

- CMV (cytomegalovirus) cultures

HUC To Do

- Notify the clinical laboratory if the test is stat (may require telephone communication).
- Write the orders on a paper Kardex or enter into computerized Kardex (if EMR c̄ CPOE is not implemented).

(Continued)

HUC To Do—Cont'd

- Order laboratory test as required (if EMR c̄ CPOE is not implemented).
- A paper requisition may be required to accompany the labeled specimen.

Serology and Immunology

Serology is the study of antibodies and antigens and is useful in detecting the presence and intensity of a current infection. It also may be useful in identifying a previous infection or exposure to an organism. Autoimmune diseases may be studied, and pretransplant and post-transplant evaluations and treatment may be provided. Tests for syphilis, rheumatoid arthritis, human immunodeficiency virus (HIV), and some influenzas, as well as tissue typing, are a few of the studies done in this area.

Antibodies, the proteins that are produced as part of an immune response, are also called *immunoglobulins*. Five main types of immunoglobulins have been identified: IgG, IgM, IgA, IgD, and IgE.

An important characteristic of antibodies is that they are often produced specifically against a particular foreign substance and are ordered in reference to that substance. Any substance that elicits an immune response is called an *antigen*. Measurement of the antibody level may be ordered as a titer. Many serologic tests are done to detect antibody levels because antibodies are usually found in the serum portion of the blood. Serologic tests can also detect the presence of antigens.

Most of these tests are done on the serum portion of a blood specimen. However, other body fluids such as spinal fluid may be tested, as may biopsy specimens and secretions from wounds. (Fasting is not required for tests performed in the Serology division of the laboratory.)

☑ *Doctors' Orders for Serology*

- Acute hepatitis panel (tests for hepatitis A, B, and C)
- ANA (antinuclear antibody) (autoimmune diseases such as SLE [systemic lupus erythematosus])
- ASO (antistreptolysin O) titer (streptococcal infection, including acute rheumatic fever)
- CEA (carcinoembryonic antigen) (liver, colon, or pancreatic cancer)
- CMV IgG and IgM (immunoglobulin G and immunoglobulin M antibodies against cytomegalovirus)
- EBV (Epstein-Barr virus) panel—determines various levels of antibodies (IgG and IgM) produced and directed against specific parts of the Epstein-Barr virus, such as viral capsid antigen (VCA) and Epstein-Barr virus nuclear antigen (EBNA)
- FTA (fluorescent treponemal antibody)—syphilis

- HB_sAg (hepatitis B surface antigen)—HB_sAg is a serum study that is done to detect the presence of hepatitis B in the blood
- HIV-1 antibody test (uses oral mucosal transudate [OMT], a serum-derived fluid that enters saliva from the gingival crevice and across oral mucosal surfaces)
- Heterophil agglutination test (infectious mononucleosis)
- RA factor (rheumatoid arthritis)
- RPR (rapid plasma reagin) test (syphilis) or VDRL (Venereal Disease Research Laboratory)
  Antibody subclasses include the following:
- IgG (immunoglobulin G)
- IgM (immunoglobulin M)
- IgD (immunoglobulin D)
- IgA (immunoglobulin A)
- IgE (immunoglobulin E)
  The method by which serology is requested may be specified. These immunoassays include the following:
- ELISA (enzyme-linked immunosorbent assay) or EIA (enzyme immunoassay)
- RIA (radioimmunoassay)
- FIA (fluorescent immunoassay)
- Comp fix (complement fixation)
- PCR (polymerase chain reaction) or RT-PCR (real-time polymerase chain reaction)
- Titer (positive or negative antibody level expressed as a ratio, e.g., 1:8)

HUC To Do

- Notify the clinical laboratory if the test is stat (may require telephone communication).
- Write the orders on a paper Kardex or enter into computerized Kardex (if EMR c̄ CPOE is not implemented).
- Order laboratory test as required (if EMR c̄ CPOE is not implemented).

Refer to Appendix E for other tests performed in the Microbiology and Serology divisions.

Blood Bank

The blood bank, which is usually a part of the clinical laboratory, has the responsibilities of typing and crossmatching patient blood, obtaining blood for transfusion, storing blood and blood components, and keeping records of transfusions and blood donors. Before whole blood, packed cells, and some other blood components are administered, the patient must have a type and crossmatch done. This is a test that determines the patient's blood type and compatibility. The four major blood groups are A, B, AB, and O.

- Patients with type A blood may receive transfusions of types A and O.
- Patients with type B may receive types B and O.
- Patients with type AB may receive types A, B, AB, and O.
- Patients with type O may receive only type O blood transfusions.
- Autologous or autotransfusion (blood transfusion using the patient's own blood)
- Donor directed or donor specific (blood of relatives or friends)
  The blood bank also performs several other blood studies, including the following:
- DAT (direct antiglobulin test) (Coombs' test)
- Direct Coombs' test (hemolytic disease of the newborn, hemolytic transfusion reactions, and acquired hemolytic anemia)
- Indirect Coombs' test (presence of antibodies to red blood cell antigens)—This test is valuable in detecting the presence of anti-Rh antibodies in the serum of a pregnant woman before the time of delivery.
- A specimen of blood is used for type and crossmatching and for type and screen. (Fasting is not required for this procedure.)

☑ Doctors' Orders for Blood Bank

- T&C for 2 U PC (type and crossmatch 2 units packed cells)
- Packed cells, 1 U (need type and crossmatching)
- Plasma, 3 U stat
- Give washed cells 1 U (need type and crossmatching)
- Cryoprecipitate 1 U
- Give 2 U of platelets (no crossmatching needed, but donor plasma and recipient RBCs should be ABO compatible)
- Normal serum albumin 5% (no crossmatching)
- T&C 6 U pc—Hold for surgery in A.M.

HUC To Do

- Notify the clinical laboratory if the test is stat (may require telephone communication).
- Write the orders on a paper Kardex or enter into computerized Kardex (if EMR c̄ CPOE is not implemented).
- Order laboratory test as required (if EMR c̄ CPOE is not implemented).
- Verify that the transfusion consent form is in the patient's chart.

Urinalysis

The Urinalysis division of the laboratory studies urine specimens for color, clarity, pH (degree of acidity or alkalinity), specific gravity (degree of concentration), protein (albumin), glucose (sugar), blood, bilirubin, and urobilinogen. The sediment is viewed microscopically for organisms, intact cells, and crystals. Urine is the specimen that is used for this test; however, the doctor may indicate that the nursing staff should follow a special procedure to obtain the specimen. (Fasting is not required for urinalysis.)

Procedures for Obtaining Urine Specimens

- Voided urine specimen (may be used for most urine tests but not collected under sterile conditions; may not be used for microbiology cultures or smears)
- Clean catch, or midstream, urine specimen (may be used for any urine test, including culture and sensitivity)
- Catheterized urine specimen (may be used for any urine test, including culture and sensitivity)

☑ *Doctors' Orders for Urinalysis*

Examples of doctors' orders for urinalysis are listed below:
- Cath UA
- Clean catch UA
- Dipstick urine for ketones
- UA today
- Urine reflex (Urine is tested in the laboratory; if certain parameters are met, the specimen will be sent to Microbiology to be cultured.)

HUC To Do

- Notify the clinical laboratory if the test is stat (may require telephone communication).
- Write the orders on a paper Kardex or enter into computerized Kardex (if EMR c̄ CPOE is not implemented).
- Order laboratory test as required (if EMR c̄ CPOE is not implemented).
- A paper requisition may be required to accompany the labeled specimen.

Nonretrievable Specimens

Some specimens are collected by the physician and may involve invasive procedures (see section on specimens). These specimens are considered "nonretrievable" because they are not easily replaced. Care should be taken in ordering tests and delivering the specimen to the clinical laboratory.

Studies Performed on Pleural Fluid

Studies are performed on pleural fluid to determine the cause and nature of pleural effusion, including hypertension, congestive heart failure (CHF), cirrhosis, infection, and neoplasm. Pleural fluid is obtained when the doctor performs a thoracentesis. The patient must sign a consent form for this procedure. (Fasting is not required for tests performed on pleural fluid.)

☑ Doctors' Orders for Pleural Fluid

Examples of doctors' orders performed on pleural fluid are listed below:
- Thoracentesis, pleural fluid to lab for LDH, glucose, and amylase
- Clinical indication (CI)—cancer
- Pleural fluid for cell count, diff
- Pleural fluid for C&S

Studies Performed on Cerebrospinal Fluid

Studies are performed on cerebrospinal fluid to identify various brain diseases, infections, and injuries. Cerebrospinal fluid (CSF) is obtained when the doctor performs a lumbar puncture. The patient must sign a consent form for this procedure. (Fasting is not required for tests performed on CSF.)

☑ Doctors' Orders for Cerebrospinal Fluid Studies

Examples of doctors' orders performed on CSF are listed below:
- Lumbar puncture, fluid to lab for cell count and diff
- CSF for serology
- CSF to lab for the following:
  tube #1—cell count, protein, and glucose;
  tube #2—AFB and fungal culture tube;
  tube #3—Gram stain

Pathology

Pathology, the study of the nature and cause of disease, involves body changes. Histology and Cytology are subdivisions of the Pathology department. A pathologist is in charge of the Pathology department.

Histology is the study of the microscopic structure of tissue. Cytology is the study of cells obtained from body tissues and fluids to determine cell type and to detect cancer or a precancerous condition.

Organs, tissues, cells, and body fluids obtained through biopsies, centesis, sternal puncture, lumbar puncture, surgery, and autopsies are studied in the Pathology department. A Pap smear is a staining method developed by Dr. George Nicolas Papanicolaou that can be performed on various types of specimens to determine the presence of cancer. However, cells from the cervix are the specimens most frequently studied (cervical smear). During a pelvic examination, the doctor may remove tissues or cells from the cervix for study.

✏ *TAKE NOTE*

Some specimens (well wrapped) may be sent by the pneumatic tube system, especially when results are needed quickly (Emergency department and Surgery). Specimens that should not be sent by the pneumatic tube system are those that have been collected through an invasive procedure, such as cerebrospinal and amniotic fluids. When blood or urine specimens are sent via the pneumatic tube system, specimens must be well wrapped and cushioned. Some facilities may have a policy not to transport *any* specimens via the pneumatic tube system because of possible loss or spilling of the specimen.

HUC To Do

- Notify the clinical laboratory if the test is stat (may require telephone communication).
- Prepare a consent form for the procedure that will be done to obtain the specimen if necessary.
- Order the appropriate sterile collection tray from Central Supply if necessary.
- Write the orders on a paper Kardex or enter into computerized Kardex (if EMR c̄ CPOE is not implemented).
- Order laboratory tests as required (if EMR c̄ CPOE is not implemented).
- A paper requisition may be required to accompany the labeled specimen.

Recording Laboratory Results

Laboratory test results are a valuable tool for the doctor in the diagnosis and treatment of patients; therefore, test result values are often communicated to the doctor before the computer report can be placed on the patient's chart. When you are calling results to a doctor's office, always have the person who is receiving the results repeat the recorded values back to you. The written report should be placed on the patient's chart in a timely manner. Accuracy in the selection of the correct patient's chart and appropriate location of information in the chart are very important.

BOX 8–5	Common Laboratory Panels

Electrolytes	BMP
Na	Na
K	K
Cl	Cl
CO_2	CO_2

(Continued)

BOX 8-5	Common Laboratory Panels—Cont'd

BUN
Creat
Gluc
Ca

Renal Panel
Na
K
Cl
CO_2
BUN
Creat
Gluc
Ca
Alb
Phosphate

CMP
Na
K
Cl
CO_2
BUN
Creatinine
Gluc
Ca
Alb
T. prot
AST
ALT
T. bili
Alk phos

Lipid Panel
Chol
Trig
LDL
HDL

Hepatic Function Panel
Albumin
T. bili
D. bili
alk phos
T. prot
AST
ALT

CBC
RBC
WBC c̄ diff
Hb
Hct
RBC indices

Acute Hepatitis Panel
HA Ab IgM
HBcAb IgM
HBsAg
Hep C Ab

Epstein-Barr Virus Panel
EBV IgM
EBV IgG
EBV EA
EBNA

Diagnostic Imaging Orders

✐ TAKE NOTE

When the EMR c̄ CPOE is implemented, the physicians' orders
are entered directly into the patient's electronic record, and
the diagnostic imaging order will automatically be sent to the

---

> ### ✎ TAKE NOTE—Cont'd
>
> Diagnostic Imaging department. The HUC may have tasks to perform, such as coordinating scheduling, ordering special diets, and so forth. An icon may indicate an HUC task, or it may follow a nurse's request. The HUC will have to communicate with the Nutritional Care department (by e-mail or telephone) when ordering a diet for a patient who has completed a diagnostic procedure that required them to be NPO (nothing by mouth). (Some hospital Nutritional Care departments require all diet orders in writing via computer.)

Many modalities, including **radiography, nuclear medicine, ultrasound, computed tomography (CT)**, and **magnetic resonance imaging (MRI)**, are available in the Diagnostic Imaging department. Diagnostic imaging procedures are performed to diagnose conditions and/or diseases (or to rule them out) and to assist the doctor in determining appropriate treatment. Additional, more detailed information regarding diagnostic imaging may be found in Chapter 15 of *LaFleur Brooks' Health Unit Coordinating*, 6th edition.

When you order the diagnostic procedure, indicate the following information about the patient:

- Reason for the procedure (clinical indication)
- Transportation required
- Whether the patient is receiving IV fluids
- Whether the patient is receiving oxygen
- Whether the patient needs isolation precautions
- If the patient has a seizure disorder
- If the patient does not speak English
- If the patient has diabetes
- If the patient is sight or hearing impaired
- If the patient is pregnant or if pregnancy test results are pending

Picture Archiving and Communication System (PACS)

A picture archiving and communication systems (PACS) consists of computers or networks that are dedicated to the storage, retrieval, distribution, and presentation of images.

Full PACS systems handle images from various modalities, such as ultrasonography, MRI, positron emission tomography, CT, endoscopy, mammography, and radiography (plain X-rays).

- PACS replaces hard copy–based means of managing medical images such as film archives. PACS provides off-site viewing and reporting (distance education, telediagnosis).

- When a study has been reported by the radiologist, the PACS can mark it as read, which avoids needless double-reading.
- Dictation of reports can be integrated into a single system. The dictated recording is automatically sent to a transcriptionist workstation for typing, but it can also be made available for access by physicians (avoiding typing delays) for urgent results, or it can be retained in case of typing error.
- The report can be attached to the images and viewable to the physician.
- Physicians at various physical locations may access the same information simultaneously.
- Global PACS networks enable images to be sent throughout the world.
- The system provides a growing cost and space advantage over film archives.
- PACS should interface with the existing hospital information system (HIS) and radiology information system (RIS). An icon that indicates a diagnostic medical image in a patient's medical record would allow the physician to view the image and the radiologist's report.
- Benefits for the doctor include faster results, ability to compare an image with a previous image (if applicable), ability to share with other physicians, and reduced risk of lost film.
- Benefits for the patient include reduction in delay of treatment, reduced risk of lost film, and protection of confidentiality.
- An added benefit is provided for the environment because X-ray photographic darkroom chemicals and toxins are eliminated from the process.

Positions Used Most Frequently in Writing X-ray Orders

- **AP position**—May be taken while the patient is standing or lying on their back (supine); machine is placed in front of the patient
- **PA position**—May be taken while the patient is standing or lying on their stomach (prone) with the X-ray machine aimed at the patient's back
- **Lateral position**—Taken with the patient standing or lying on their side
- **Oblique position**—Taken with the patient standing or lying halfway on their side in the AP or PA position
- **Decubitus position**—In this view, the patient is lying on their side with the X-ray beam positioned horizontally.

Informed Consent Forms

Diagnostic imaging procedures that are invasive—those that require the injection of contrast medium—require the patient to sign a consent form after they have been informed of procedures, risks, alternatives, outcomes, and so forth. Special invasive X-ray procedures require a signed consent form because iodinated contrast medium is used. Other diagnostic imaging procedures that require a consent form may vary among health care facilities.

Types of contrast media include the following:

- Barium preparations
- Organic iodine compounds
- Water
- Air
- Gas
- Radiopharmaceuticals (nuclear medicine)

Examples of routine preparations may include the following:

- Diet orders (including fat free, cl liq, or NPO 2400)
- Cleansing enemas
- Cathartics (laxatives)—citrate of mag, GoLytely, Dulcolax, or Fleet

Sequencing

Typical guidelines for scheduling X-ray studies include the following:

- Order X-ray studies of the lower spine and pelvis first, before a barium enema or an upper gastrointestinal study is done. The presence of barium in specific parts of the body may obscure the portion of the body that is being studied.
- Abdominal studies with ultrasound or CT should precede studies in which barium is used.
- Liver and bone scans and nuclear medicine studies may conflict with barium studies and should be done first.
- Three X-ray studies that require contrast media are frequently ordered at the same time for diagnostic reasons. Only one or sometimes two can be done on the same day; thus, these studies may have to be scheduled 3 or more days in advance.
- The order of scheduling is listed below:
  - Intravenous urogram (IVU)—special invasive procedures
  - Barium enema (BE)
  - Upper gastrointestinal (UGI) or UGI and small bowel follow-through (SBFT)

Overview of Radiology

X-rays, similar to visible light, are a form of electromagnetic radiation. Created images are recorded with a computer or special film.

Examples of Radiology Procedures That Do Not Require Preparation or Contrast Media

Procedures	Purpose
Skeletal X-rays	Diagnose abnormalities, disease, fractures of bones

(Continued)

Overview of Radiology—Cont'd

Chest PA and LAT	Evaluate for surgery; diagnose obstructions, abnormalities, and disease
KUB	Diagnoses abnormalities, obstruction, disease within the abdomen (also called a flat plate of abdomen)
SNAT series	Detects abuse (child or adult) (x-ray of long bones, skull, and spine)
Bone age study	Determines child development/growth (x-ray of left wrist)

Examples of Radiology Procedures That Do Require Preparation or Contrast Media

Procedures	Purpose
BE or ulcerative colitis	Identifies disease of the large intestine (e.g., diverticula, cancer)
IVU (IVP)	Diagnoses abnormalities, stricture, urinary system disease
UGI	Detects hiatal hernia, strictures, ulcers, and tumors

BE, Barium enema; IVP, intravenous pyelogram; IVU, intravenous urogram; KUB, kidneys, ureters, and bladder; LAT, lateral; PA, posteroanterior; SNAT, suspected nonaccidental trauma; UGI, upper gastrointestinal.

Overview of Special Invasive X-ray Procedures

Special invasive X-ray procedures are performed under the direction of the radiologist or a surgeon with a radiologist present. Contrast is given and a signed consent is required for special procedures. On-call medication may or may not be ordered by the patient's doctor.

Examples of Special Invasive X-ray Procedures

Procedure	Purpose
Arthrogram	Detects trauma, such as bone chips or torn ligaments, from an injury
Angiogram	Diagnoses vascular aneurysms, malformations, occluded or leaking blood vessels
Voiding cystourethrogram	Demonstrates bladder and urethral strictures
Venogram	Evaluates veins before and after bypass surgery and for obstruction
Spinal myelogram	Detects herniated disks, tumors, and spinal nerve root injuries

Overview of Special Invasive X-ray Procedures—Cont'd

Hysterosalpingogram   Confirms abnormalities, such as adhesions and fistulas, when used in fertility studies

Lymphangiogram   Identifies metastatic cancer in lymph nodes; evaluates chemotherapy treatment

Overview of Computed Tomography

Computed tomography uses a type of ionizing radiation to provide a computerized image that can generate multidimensional sections (slices) of tissue. Contrast media may or may not be used.

Examples of CT Procedures

Procedure	Purpose
CT of head c̄ DSA	To evaluate postoperatively (e.g., endarterectomy); detects any cerebrovascular abnormality
Chest CT	Detects lung changes, pneumonia, cancer, pulmonary embolism, aortic dissection, and other conditions
Abdominal CT	Detects cancer, aortic aneurysm, bowel obstruction, and other conditions
Head CT	Diagnoses brain tumor, infarction, bleeding hematoma
LS spine CT	Confirms spinal stenosis and changes in disks and vertebrae; confirms spinal infection

DSA, Digital subtraction angiograpzhy; LS, lumbosacral.

Overview of Ultrasound (Sonography)

Ultrasonography, also called *sonography* or *echography*, uses high-frequency sound waves to create an image of body organs. Female pelvic ultrasound would require a full bladder.

(Continued)

Overview of Ultrasound (Sonography)—Cont'd

Examples of Ultrasound Procedures

Procedure	Purpose
Gallbladder	Diagnoses cholelithiasis, cholecystitis; identifies obstructive jaundice
Pelvis	Identifies ovarian cancer, other disorders; identifies ectopic pregnancy, multiple births, fetal abnormalities
Abdomen	Detects liver cysts, abscesses, hematomas, tumors

Ultrasound is also useful in examining other internal organs, including but not limited to, kidneys, heart and blood vessels, bladder, uterus, ovaries, unborn child (fetus) in pregnant patients, eyes, thyroid and parathyroid glands, and scrotum (testicles).

Overview of Magnetic Resonance Imaging

Magnetic resonance imaging is a technique that is used for viewing the interior of the body with the use of a powerful magnetic field, radio waves, and a computer to produce images of body structures. Contrast media may or may not be used. A completed interview form is required.

Examples of MRI Procedures

Procedure	Purpose
MRI	Diagnoses internal injuries, conditions, disease in any body part to monitor effects of medications and treatments inside the body

MRI contraindications exist for patients with the following:

*Pacemaker	*Implanted port device
*Neurostimulator	*Intrauterine device (IUD)
Insulin pump	Older metal plates, pins, screws, or surgical staples
Ear implant	Older metal clips from aneurysm repair
Metal clips in eyes	Retained bullets
Pregnancy	Any other large metal objects implanted in the body (tooth fillings and braces are usually not a problem)

Note: Only ferrous (iron-based) devices are attracted by magnet. Today, 99.9% of devices are safe for MRI. (The physician would have to be consulted.)

Overview of Nuclear Medicine

Nuclear imaging examines organ function and structure, whereas diagnostic radiology is based on anatomy. Contrast agents are used.

Overview of Nuclear Medicine—Cont'd

Examples of Nuclear Imaging Procedures

Procedure	Purpose
Lung perfusion	Diagnoses pulmonary embolism
Liver and spleen scan	Evaluates injury to spleen, chronic hepatitis, metastatic processes
Renal scan	Examines kidneys and detects any abnormalities such as tumors or obstruction of renal blood flow
Thyroid scan	Evaluates thyroid function
Bone scan	Evaluates any degenerative and/or arthritic changes in joints; detects bone diseases and tumors; determines cause of bone pain or inflammation
Gallium scan	Diagnoses active infectious, inflammatory disease; tumors; and abscesses
Brain scan	Investigates problems within and blood circulation to the brain
Breast scan	Used with mammograms to locate cancerous breast tissue
OctreoScan	Finds primary and metastatic neuroendocrine tumors
HIDA scan (cholescintigraphy)	Diagnoses bile duct obstruction, gallbladder disease, bile leaks
NeutroSpec scanning	Identifies abdominal, chest, and deep space infections otherwise not clinically apparent
PET scan	Obtains information about blood flow to the myocardium, metabolism, glucose utilization, or schizophrenia
Scrotal nuclear imaging	Differentiates testicular torsion from other causes of pain
WBC scan	Identifies, localizes occult inflammation or infection

Heart Scans

Myocardial perfusion	Identifies ischemic or infarcted heart muscle
Myocardial function (MUGA)	Most accurate method used to determine cardiac ejection fraction
Cardiac flow	Performed in children with suspected cardiac anomalies
Nuclear ventriculography	Evaluates muscle wall activity
Exercise stress test	Evaluates muscle wall activity during stress (physical or chemical)

HIDA, Hepatobiliary iminodiacetic acid scan; MUGA, multiple gated acquisition scan; PET, positron emission tomography; WBC, white blood cell.

HUC To Do

- Some computer systems will automatically print directions for preparations when a procedure is entered into the computer.
- Some hospitals have a file box with routine preparations printed out on cards that may be placed in the patient's Kardex or given to the nurse.
- Send the order to the appropriate division of the Diagnostic Imaging department (if EMR c̄ CPOE is not implemented).
- Send nutritional care order to the Nutritional Care department (NPO 2400, etc.) (if EMR c̄ CPOE is not implemented).
- Prepare a consent form for patients who are about to undergo a special procedure.
- Because barium would obscure the view of certain organs, it is important to order procedures with barium used last.
- When you are transcribing MRI orders, prepare an interview form for the nurse to complete before sending the patient for an MRI. This form should list any contraindications that may prevent the patient from having the procedure.
- Send/fax pharmacy copies to the pharmacy (if EMR c̄ CPOE is not implemented).
- Write orders on a paper Kardex or enter into computerized Kardex (if EMR c̄ CPOE is not implemented).

Other Diagnostic Studies

Overview of Neurology Department Tests

Neurologic tests include those related to the function of the nervous system (brain and spinal cord). In smaller facilities, electroencephalography (EEG) may be the only neurodiagnostic test that is performed.

Tests Performed by Neurology
- Electroencephalography (EEG)
- Visual-evoked potential (VEP)
- Brainstem auditory-evoked response (BAER) or auditory brainstem-evoked potential (ABEP)
- Somatosensory-evoked potential (SEP)
- Caloric study (oculovestibular reflex study)
- Electronystagmography (ENG) (electrooculography)
- Electromyography (EMG)
- Electroneurography (nerve conduction studies)

HUC To Do

- Send the order to the Neurology department (if EMR c̄ CPOE is not implemented).
- A list of neurologic medications the patient is taking may be required when these procedures are ordered.

Overview of Cardiovascular Diagnostic Tests

The results of electrodiagnostic tests and other cardiovascular studies aid the physician in making a diagnosis and prescribing treatment.

Noninvasive Cardiovascular Tests

- Electrocardiogram (EKG or ECG)
- Rhythm strip
- Impedance cardiography (IPG)
- Holter monitor
- Cardiac stress test (exercise EKG or treadmill stress test)
- Thallium or sestamibi stress test (discussed in Chapter 15, p. 303)
- Echocardiogram
- Transesophageal echocardiogram
- Plethysmography vascular studies
- Vascular ultrasound studies
- Vascular duplex scans

Invasive Cardiovascular Tests (usually requiring sedation of the patient)

- Electrophysiologic study (EPS)
- Cardiac catheterization (coronary angiography, angiocardiography, ventriculography)—*consent required; medical procedures (angioplasty with stents or a coronary artery bypass graft [CABG]) may be performed during or scheduled after the catheterization to correct blocked blood vessels*
- Swan-Ganz catheter insertion

HUC To Do

- Send the order to the Cardiovascular department (if EMR c̄ CPOE is not implemented).
- A list of cardiovascular medications the patient is taking may be required when these procedures are ordered.
- Write orders on a paper Kardex or enter into computerized Kardex (if EMR c̄ CPOE is not implemented).

Overview of Endoscopies

All endoscopies (procedures performed to visualize and examine a body cavity or hollow organ) require signed consent. Biopsies are sometimes performed during endoscopic procedures. Preparations vary depending on the procedure, the ordering doctor, and whether general anesthesia is used. NPO (nothing by mouth) 2400 hours usually is required for all endoscopies.

Endoscopy	Area of Visualization	Prep
Arthroscopy	Joints	NPO
Bronchoscopy	Larynx, trachea, bronchi, alveoli	NPO
Colonoscopy	Rectum, colon	Yes
Colposcopy	Vagina, cervix	No
Cystoscopy	Urethra, bladder, ureters, prostate (male)	Yes
Enteroscopy	Upper colon, small intestines	Yes
Endourology	Bladder and urethra	No
Endoscopic retrograde cholangiopancreatography	Pancreatic and biliary ducts	NPO
Esophagogastroduodenoscopy	Esophagus, stomach, duodenum	Yes
Fetoscopy	Fetus	No
Gastroscopy	Stomach	NPO
Hysteroscopy	Uterus	NPO
Laparoscopy	Abdominal cavity	Yes
Mediastinoscopy	Mediastinal lymph nodes	NPO
Sigmoidoscopy	Sigmoid colon	Yes
Sinus endoscopy	Sinus cavities	NPO
Thoracoscopy	Pleura, lung	NPO

HUC To Do

- Send the order to the Endoscopy department (if EMR c̄ CPOE is not implemented).
- Send nutritional care orders to the Nutritional Care department (if EMR c̄ CPOE is not implemented).
- Prepare a consent form.
- Write orders on a paper Kardex or enter into computerized Kardex (if EMR c̄ CPOE is not implemented).

Overview of Gastrointestinal Studies

Some gastrointestinal (GI) studies are performed in the endoscopy department, usually on an outpatient basis; others may be performed at the bedside by the nurse. Specimens collected by the nurse are sent to the hospital clinical laboratory for study, or they may be sent to a private laboratory.

- **Gastric analysis**—Measures the stomach's secretion of hydrochloric acid and pepsin and evaluates stomach and duodenal ulcers.
- **Esophageal manometry (esophageal function study, esophageal motility study)**—Identifies and documents disease severity that affects the swallowing function of the esophagus. Also documents and quantifies gastroesophageal reflux.
- **Secretin test**—Evaluates pancreatic function after hormone secretin stimulation; measures volume and bicarbonate concentration of pancreatic secretions; lower than normal volume suggests an obstructing malignancy or cystic fibrosis.

Overview of the Cardiopulmonary (Respriratory Care) Department (Diagnostics)

The Cardiopulmonary (Respiratory Care) department evaluates, treats, and cares for patients with breathing or other cardiopulmonary disorders. The Cardiopulmonary (Respiratory Care) department also may perform presurgical evaluations.

Diagnostic Tests Performed by the Cardiopulmonary (Respiratory Care) Department

- **Oximetry (pulse oximetry, ear oximetry, oxygen saturation)**—Monitors arterial oxygen saturation levels (SaO_2) in patients at risk for hypoxemia. A monitoring probe or sensor is clipped to the finger or the ear.
- **Arterial blood gases (ABGs)**—Monitors patients on ventilators, critically ill nonventilator patients; establishes preoperative baseline parameters, regulates electrolyte therapy. A point-of-care (POC) ABG portable device may be used to perform ABG and pH measurements.
- **Capillary blood gases (CBGs)**—Performed primarily on infants. Blood is obtained from the infant's capillary arterial vessel, usually from the heel, by the respiratory care technician.
- **Pulmonary function tests (PFTs)**—Detect abnormalities in respiratory function and determine the extent of pulmonary abnormality. Tests usually include spirometry, measurement of air flow rates, and calculation of lung volumes and capacities.

(Continued)

Overview of the Cardiopulmonary (Respriratory Care) Department (Diagnostics)—Cont'd

- **Spirometry**—Determines air volumes and air flow rates. Air flow rates provide information about airway obstruction. The patient breathes through a sterile mouthpiece into a spirometer, inhaling as deeply as possible and then forcibly exhaling as much air as possible. The test may be repeated with the use of bronchodilators if values are deficient. The doctor may order a prebronchodilator and a postbronchodilator spirometry study.

HUC To Do

- Send orders to the Cardiopulmonary (Respiratory Care) department (if EMR c̄ CPOE is not implemented).
- Write orders on a paper Kardex or enter into computerized Kardex (if EMR c̄ CPOE is not implemented).
- When ordering ABGs, note whether the patient is on room air or on oxygen and the number of liters. If anticoagulants are being administered to the patient, the medications (e.g., enoxaparin [Lovenox], heparin [Hepalean], warfarin [Coumadin]) may have to be noted as well. The arterial blood specimen needs to be placed on ice immediately and taken to the pulmonary laboratory for analysis.

✐ TAKE NOTE

Normal pH Values
Adult/Child: 7.35 to 7.45
Newborn: 7.32 to 7.49
2 months to 2 years: 7.34 to 7.46
pH (venous): 7.31 to 7.41

Critical Values
pH: <7.25 to >7.55
PCO_2: <20, >60
HCO_3: <15, >40
PO_2: <40
O_2 saturation: 75% or lower
Base/Excess: + mEq/L

Sleep Studies

Sleep studies are ordered for patients who snore excessively; experience narcolepsy, excessive daytime sleeping, or insomnia; or have motor spasms while sleeping, as well as for patients with documented cardiac rhythm disturbances limited to sleep time. Several tests, including EKG, EEG, EMG, air flow, and oximetry, are included in a sleep study.

Inductive plethysmography, a noninvasive study that measures the patient's respiratory function, can differentiate central apnea from obstructive sleep apnea during a sleep study. Most sleep studies are performed on an outpatient basis.

HUC To Do

- Send order to the Sleep Study department (if EMR c̄ CPOE is not implemented).
- Write orders on a paper Kardex or enter into computerized Kardex (if EMR c̄ CPOE is not implemented).

Treatment Orders

Overview of Cardiovascular Treatment

Patients with cardiovascular conditions may be treated with medication and/or surgery and/or placement of a pacemaker.

- **Insertion of a cardiac pacemaker**—Usually used to correct bradycardia. A pacemaker may be permanent or temporary, may emit the stimulus at a constant and fixed rate, or may fire only on demand.
- **Insertion of an implantable cardioverter-defibrillator (ICD)**—An electronic device that monitors and restores proper rhythm when the heart begins to beat rapidly (tachycardia) or erratically by sending low-energy shocks to the heart.
- **Angioplasty (balloon angioplasty, coronary angioplasty, coronary artery angioplasty, cardiac angioplasty, percutaneous transluminal coronary angioplasty [PTCA], heart artery dilatation)**—Procedure in which a balloon is used to open narrowed or blocked blood vessels of the heart (coronary arteries). Although it is an invasive procedure and a consent is required, it is not considered to be a type of surgery. An angioplasty is usually performed during a heart catheterization, when it is deemed necessary.
- **Stent**—Most always also placed at the site of a narrowing or blockage to keep the artery open. An intraluminal coronary artery stent is a small, self-expanding, metal mesh tube placed inside a coronary artery after balloon angioplasty to prevent the artery from re-closing. A drug-eluting stent is coated with medicine (sirolimus or paclitaxel) to further prevent the arteries from re-closing. Similar to other coronary stents, it is left permanently in the artery (Fig. 8-3).
- **Rotational arthrectomy**—In a small number of cases, a special catheter with a small, diamond tip is used to drill through hard plaque and calcium that are causing the blockage.

(Continued)

Overview of Cardiovascular Treatment—Cont'd

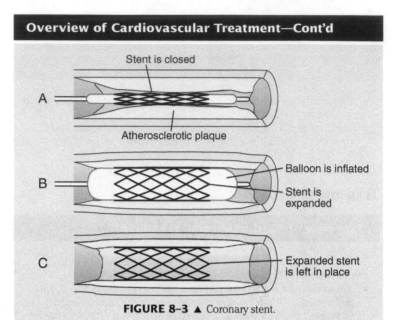

Stent is closed

A

Atherosclerotic plaque

Balloon is inflated

B

Stent is expanded

C

Expanded stent is left in place

FIGURE 8–3 ▲ Coronary stent.

- **Coronary artery bypass graft (CABG) (referred to as a "cabbage")**—Surgical treatment for blocked arteries when they are too severely blocked to be treated with angioplasty. Heart bypass surgery creates a detour or "bypass" around the blocked part of a coronary artery to restore the blood supply to the heart muscle (Fig. 8-4).
- **Artery and vein grafts**—The saphenous vein, a vein from the leg, may be used for the bypass. An incision is made in the leg and the vein is removed. The vein is located on the inside of the leg, running from the ankle to the groin. The internal mammary artery (IMA) can also be used as the graft. The IMA has the advantage of staying open for many more years than the vein grafts, but in some situations, it cannot be used. Other arteries are also now being used in bypass surgery, the most common being the radial artery (one of two arteries that supply the hand with blood). It usually can be removed from the arm without impairment of blood supply to the hand. Traditionally, the patient is connected to the heart-lung machine, or the bypass pump, which adds oxygen to the blood and circulates blood to other parts of the body during the surgery.
- **Other surgical techniques (off-pump coronary artery bypass [OPCAB])**—Allow the bypass to be created while the heart is still beating. Another alternative is smaller incisions that avoid splitting the breastbone, referred to as minimally-invasive direct coronary artery bypass (MIDCAB).

Overview of Cardiovascular Treatment—Cont'd

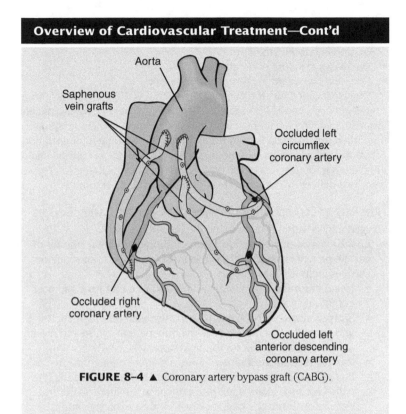

FIGURE 8–4 ▲ Coronary artery bypass graft (CABG).

Coronary bypass surgery now can be performed with the aid of a robot, which allows the surgeon to perform the operation without even being in the same room as the patient. A surgical consent form is required, and the patient is admitted to the coronary intensive care unit after surgery.

📝 *TAKE NOTE*

The consent form for heart catheterization will usually include all possible corrective options, so the surgeon can proceed with the procedure or surgery as required.

Overview of Cardiopulmonary (Respiratory Care) Treatments

The Cardiopulmonary (Respiratory Care) department performs treatments to maintain or improve the function of the respiratory system. These treatments are usually performed at the patient's bedside by a respiratory therapist.

Oxygen Therapy

- Treats hypoxemia (abnormal deficiency in the concentration of oxygen in arterial blood).
- Decreases the work of breathing.
- Decreases myocardial (heart muscle) work.

Oxygen is piped into the patient's room via a wall outlet and is administered under pressure. A portable oxygen tank may be used when a patient is transported. Oxygen therapy may have a drying effect on the respiratory tract; therefore, oxygen is commonly humidified during administration. An oxygen order specifies the amount of oxygen (flow rate or concentration) the patient is to receive and the type of delivery device that is to be used (mode of delivery). The flow rate is ordered in liters per minute.

Flow Rate or Concentration of Oxygen and Administration Devices

Oxygen may be administered using the following:

- **Low-flow systems**—Provide only a portion of the total amount of gas the patient is breathing; the rest must be added from room air
  Devices include the following:
  - **Nasal cannula**—Frequently referred to as **nasal prongs;** most commonly used.
  - **Simple mask**—Device that is generally used for emergencies and short-term therapies; it fits over the patient's nose and mouth and acts as a reservoir for the next breath.
  - **Partial rebreathing mask**—Uses a simple mask connected to a bag reservoir with no valve between the bag and the mask. It is called a *partial rebreathing mask* because the first one third of exhalation enters the bag, mixes with source oxygen, and is consumed during the next inhalation.
  - **Nonrebreathing mask**—Designed to fit over the patient's nose and mouth as the simple oxygen mask does; however, a 500 to 1000-mL plastic bag is added to the mask, which includes a series of one-way valves that permit the reservoir bag to fill only with pure oxygen.
- **High-flow systems**—Provide enough gas flow to meet all of the patient's ventilatory demands
  Devices include the following:
  - **Jet mixing mask**, also referred to as a **Venti mask**—Delivers a total high flow by mixing oxygen with room air. The mask takes pure oxygen from the flow meter and mixes it with a certain proportion of room air to deliver a higher concentration of oxygen.
  - **Large-volume nebulizer**—Another example of a high-flow system. This device works much like the jet mixing mask does, but it also provides bland (nonmedicated) aerosol therapy and can be connected to a variety of devices, including an aerosol mask, a face tent for patients with facial burns or those who cannot tolerate a mask, a T-piece or Briggs adapter for intubated patients, or a tracheostomy mask (collar) for patients with a tracheostomy.

Aerosol Treatments

Delivery devices include the following:

- **Metered-dose inhaler (MDI)**—Small, portable aerosol canisters filled with medication; the most common type of aerosol treatment. Usually, metered-dose inhalers are self-administered and require patient education and cooperation.
- **Small-volume nebulizer (SVN) (handheld nebulizer [HHN])**— Treatments last between 8 and 12 minutes and allow for numerous breaths to administer the medication. Small-volume nebulizers also may be called *spontaneous nebulizer treatments* or *jet nebulizer treatments*, or they may be referred to by the brand name of the nebulizer device.
- **Dry powder inhaler (DPI)**—Devices that deliver the drug in powder form to be delivered into the lungs for absorption. Usually, dry powder inhalers are self-administered and require patient education and cooperation.
- **Hypertonic ultrasonic nebulizer (USN)**—Often is used with hypertonic solution to induce a sputum specimen. A Lukens sputum trap is often used by a respiratory therapist to collect a sterile induced sputum specimen.
- **Intermittent positive-pressure breathing (IPPB)**—A technique that is used to provide short-term or intermittent mechanical ventilation for the purpose of augmenting lung expansion, delivering aerosol medication, clearing retained secretions, or assisting ventilation. An IPPB treatment is usually administered with a pneumatically-driven, pressure-triggered, and pressure-cycled ventilator.

Types of Aerosolized Drugs

- **Nasal decongestants**—Found primarily as over-the-counter (OTC) squeeze bottles that are sprayed into nostrils. These drugs are classified as vasoconstrictors. An example of a nasal decongestant is Neo-Synephrine.
- **Bronchodilators**—Enlarge the diameter of the airway, most often by relaxing the smooth muscle that surrounds the airways. Examples of bronchodilators include Ventolin, Atrovent, Maxair, and Serevent.
- **Antiasthmatics**—A relatively new category of drugs that desensitize the allergic response to prevent or decrease the incidence of asthma. Examples of antiasthmatics include cromolyn sodium and nedocromil sodium.
- **Corticosteroids**—Used in moderate and severe asthma attacks to reduce the inflammatory response within the lung. They are also used on a standing basis to prevent inflammation. Examples of corticosteroids include Pulmicort, Vanceril, Flovent, and Azmacort.
- **Mucolytics**—Break down secretions within the lungs to make it easier to expectorate and clear the lungs. Examples of mucolytics include Pulmozyme and Mucomyst.

- **Antimicrobials**—Aerosolized antibiotics and antiviral agents that fight both bacterial and viral infections involving the respiratory system. Examples of antimicrobials include gentamicin, tobramycin, amphotericin B, ribavirin, and pentamidine.

Other Respiratory Treatments

- **Incentive spirometry (IS)**—Also known as sustained maximal inspiration (SMI); often used postoperatively to encourage and reinforce the patient to take protracted, slow, deep breaths. The benefits of IS include improving inspiratory muscle performance and reestablishing or simulating the normal pattern of pulmonary hyperinflation.
- **Chest percussion therapy (CPT)**—Used to loosen secretions in the area underlying the percussion through air pressure that is generated by the cupped hand on the chest wall. This treatment usually is provided in conjunction with postural drainage, a treatment of patient positioning designed to remove secretions from the lung.
- **Mechanical ventilator**—Chiefly used in intensive care medicine, home care, emergency medicine (as stand-alone units), and anesthesia as a component of an anesthesia machine. Mechanical ventilation is indicated when the patient's spontaneous ventilation is inadequate to maintain life. It is also indicated to prevent imminent collapse of other physiologic functions or ineffective gas exchange in the lungs. **Weaning** is a term that is used to describe the gradual removal of mechanical ventilation from a patient. ABG will be ordered at intervals to monitor ventilator settings. Extubation orders will be written when the patient is to be removed from the ventilator. Postextubation orders will be written after the patient has been removed from the ventilator to monitor their respiratory status. Settings for a mechanical ventilator include the following:
- **Chronic obstructive pulmonary disease (COPD)**—initial ventilator settings
  - **Noninvasive**
  - **Mode**—Assist/control (pressure) or pressure support
  - **Tidal volume (TV)**—6 to 8 mL/kg ideal body weight (IBW)
  - **Positive end-expiratory pressure (PEEP)**—3 to 8 cm H_2O
  - **Ventilating pressure**—8 to 12 cm H_2O
  - **Inspiratory time**—<1.0 second
  - **Fraction of inspired oxygen (F_iO_2)**—To maintain partial pressure of oxygen in arterial blood (PaO_2) >60 mm Hg
  - **Backup rate**—8 to 10, actual patient's rate determines baseline pressure of carbon dioxide ($PaCO_2$)
- **Noninvasive positive-pressure ventilation (NIPPV)**—The application of positive pressure by noninvasive means to patients

with acute or chronic respiratory failure or to wean patients from ventilatory support

Traction

Traction is the process of putting a limb, bone, or group of muscles under tension by means of weights and pulleys to align or immobilize, to reduce muscle spasm, or to relieve pressure on the muscle. This approach is used to treat fractures, dislocations, and long-duration muscle spasms, and to prevent or correct deformities. Traction can be used on a short or long-term basis.

Two basic types of traction used in orthopedics for the treatment of fractured bones and the correction of orthopedic abnormalities include the following:

- **Skin traction** applies pull to an affected body structure with the use of straps attached to the skin surrounding the structure. Two types of skin traction include adhesive and nonadhesive skin traction.
  Examples of skin traction orders are listed here:
  - Skin traction 5 lb to lt arm
  - Skin traction 7 lb to pelvis
  - Left unilateral Buck's skin traction 5 lb
  - Russell's traction rt leg c̄ 10# weight
- **Skeletal traction** is applied to the affected structure by a metal pin or wire inserted into the structure and attached to traction ropes. Skeletal traction is often used when continuous traction is desired to immobilize, position, and align a fractured bone properly during the healing process.
  Examples of skeletal traction orders are listed here:
  - Cervical traction c̄ Crutchfield tongs
  - Thomas leg splint c̄ Steinmann pin 20 lb of traction

Apparatus Setup

Bed

The apparatus attached to the patient's bed may include pulleys, rope, weights, and metal bars. The weights (metal disks or sandbags) provide the "pull" to a part of the body. The pulleys, rope, and metal bars are assembled to suspend the weights. It is usually the responsibility of the nurse or an orthopedic technician to attach the traction apparatus to the bed. Physical Therapy department personnel may assist with setting up traction equipment in smaller hospitals.

Overhead Frame and Trapeze Bar

An overhead frame and trapeze **(trapeze bar)** is used to help the patient move and support weight during transfer or position change. It also may aid in strengthening the upper extremities.

Patient

The apparatus that is attached to the patient may be an external attachment such as a halter, belt, or boot, or an internal attachment such as a pin, tongs, or wires placed directly into the bone by the surgeon. The external apparatus is applied to the patient by the nursing staff; sometimes the HUC must order the necessary supplies from the CSD.

Although the types of supplies used vary among hospitals, moleskin tape, slings, and sandbags are commonly requisitioned from the CSD.

HUC To Do

- Order supplies/equipment as required from the CSD or from Ortho Tech.
- Notify the patient's nurse of the orders.
- Write orders on a paper Kardex or enter into computerized Kardex (if EMR c̄ CPOE is not implemented).

Physical Medicine and Rehabilitation

Most hospitals have a Physical Medicine department that provides physical therapy, occupational therapy, and speech therapy.

Physical Therapy

Physical therapy is the division of the Physical Medicine department in the hospital that treats patients to improve and restore their functional mobility through methods such as gait training, exercise, water therapy, and heat and ice treatments. Patients include those injured in accidents, sports, or work-related activities. Children affected by cerebral palsy and muscular dystrophy are assisted toward normal physical development through physical therapy. Individuals who have strokes, spinal cord injuries, and amputations are assisted back to their highest level of physical function through therapy.

☑️ *Doctors' Orders for Physical Therapy*

Hydrotherapy
- *Hubbard tank*—Used for underwater exercises and for cleansing wounds and burns; hydrotherapy treatments may be ordered to be done with a sterile solution
- *Whirlpool bath left lower extremity (LLE) bid*—Smaller than the Hubbard tank and used for the same purposes

Exercises

Passive

- Active assistive
- Progressive
- Resistive
- Muscle reeducation
- Coordination
- Relaxation
- Range of motion (ROM)
- Passive range of motion (PROM)
- T-band exercises
- Codman's exercises

Isometrics

- Joint mobilization
- Walker train
- PT to evaluate and treat
- ACL (anterior cruciate ligament) protocol
- BKA (below the knee amputation) protocol
- THA (total hip arthroplasty) and TKA (total knee arthroplasty) protocols
- Transfer training, wheelchair mobility
- Gait training with a walker
- Crutch walking NWB (non–weight bearing) daily
- CPM (continuous passive motion)

Heat and Cold Orders

- Ultrasound and massage
- Hydrocollator packs or hot packs
- Ice or cold packs

Pain Relief Orders

- Postop TENS (transcutaneous electrical nerve stimulation)

Occupational Therapy

Occupational therapy (OT) is the division of the Physical Medicine department in the hospital that works in conjunction with other health team members toward rehabilitation of patients to return them to the greatest possible functional independence. Creative, manual, recreational, and prevocational assessments are examples of activities used in rehabilitation of the patient.

✐ TAKE NOTE

Examples of basic skills to be achieved as a result of occupational therapy include toileting, bathing and dressing, cooking, and feeding oneself.

☑ *Doctors' Orders for Occupational Therapy*

- OT for evaluation and treatment
- ADL (activities of daily living) training
- Supply and train in adaptive equipment
- OT to increase mobility

HUC To Do

- Send orders to the Physical Medicine department (PT, OT, or speech therapy) (if EMR c̄ CPOE is not implemented).
- Write orders on a paper Kardex or enter into computerized Kardex (if EMR c̄ CPOE is not implemented).

Wound Care Department/Clinic

Hyperbaric Oxygen Therapy (HBOT)

- Treatment in which the patient breathes 100% oxygen while in an enclosed system that is pressurized to greater than normal atmospheric pressure (3 times normal); this is called a hyperbaric chamber.
- Hyperbaric oxygen therapy delivers oxygen quickly, systemically, and in high concentrations to injured areas.
- The increased pressure changes the normal cellular respiration process and causes oxygen to dissolve in the plasma. This stimulates the growth of new blood vessels and a substantial increase in tissue oxygenation that can arrest certain types of infections and enhance wound healing.
- Hyperbaric oxygen therapy generally is administered on an outpatient basis.

Dialysis

The kidneys are essential organs in the removal of toxic wastes from the blood. When the kidneys fail to remove those wastes, medical intervention is necessary to sustain life. The kidneys may fail temporarily (acute renal failure), or they may be permanently damaged and become nonfunctional (chronic renal failure and end-stage renal disease [ESRD]).

Two main types of dialysis are used:
- **Hemodialysis** (also called *extracorporeal dialysis*) is the removal of waste products from the blood with the use of a machine through which the blood flows. This is regularly performed in a special outpatient dialysis facility and is commonly done for 3 to 4-hour periods 3 days a week. For the hospitalized patient, hemodialysis is usually performed in a special unit in the hospital. If the patient is too ill to be moved, a portable hemodialysis machine may be used.

■ **Peritoneal dialysis** is the introduction of a fluid (dialyzing fluid) into the abdominal cavity that then absorbs the wastes from the blood through the lining of the abdominal cavity, or peritoneum. The dialysate is then emptied from the abdominal cavity. This type of dialysis allows a greater level of freedom for the patient because this fluid transfer may be performed outside of any health care facility. Some variations in peritoneal dialysis include **continuous ambulatory peritoneal dialysis (CAPD)**, **continuous cycling peritoneal dialysis (CCPD)**, and **intermittent peritoneal dialysis (IPD)**.

Radiation Treatments

The area in the hospital where radiation therapy is performed may be a division of the Diagnostic Imaging department, or it may be a totally separate department.

Many patients undergoing radiation therapies are outpatients. However, the HUC may be called upon to schedule an appointment for an inpatient who requires treatment for a malignant neoplasm (cancer). Many hospitals require that units use a requisition form; others may schedule an appointment by telephone. After the initial visit, Radiation Therapy usually notifies the nursing unit of the patient's treatment schedule.

Miscellaneous Orders
Consultation Orders

Calling a Consult

The following information should be communicated to the consulting doctor's office:
■ Hospital name
■ Patient's name and age
■ Patient's location (unit and room number)
■ Name of the doctor requesting the consultation
■ Patient's diagnosis
■ Urgency of consultation and any additional information provided in the order
■ Patient's insurance information located on the patient's face sheet

HUC To Do

■ Notify the consulting doctor's office of the order.
■ Prepare for the call to the doctor's office or answering service by writing the doctor's telephone number on a note pad and having the patient's chart close by so you have access to any additional requested information.

(Continued)

HUC To Do—Cont'd

- Document the time of notification and the name or operator number of the person (answering service) spoken to. Write this information next to the doctor's order on the doctors' order sheet with your initials.

Note: Some hospitals may have a policy requiring the requesting doctor to notify the specialist so patient history and additional information may be provided.

Typed consultation reports sent to the unit or brought in by the patient's doctor are filed in the patient's paper chart. When the EMR c̄ CPOE is implemented, the physician may enter findings and recommendations directly into the patient's EMR via computer, or reports brought from a doctor's office may be scanned into the patient's EMR. The consulting doctor will usually take a copy of the patient's face sheet back to their office for billing purposes.

Health Information Management Orders

The Health Information Management Services or department (HIMS), also called Medical Records or Health Records, stores the charts of patients who have been treated at the health care facility in the past.

Ordering and Obtaining Patient Health Records

Records from recent hospital admissions will be sent to the unit upon readmission of a patient when requested by the patient's doctor. HIMS personnel will send the old records or will print a hard copy if the record has been microfilmed. The doctor may also request medical records from the patient's previous stay in another hospital. The patient must give written permission for release of the information from one hospital to another. While old records are on the nursing unit, they are labeled with the patient's identification and stored in a designated area, rather than in the current patient's chart holder.

HUC To Do

- Send or call the order to HIMS.
- To transcribe a doctors' order to obtain health records from another hospital, place a call to the HIMS of the other hospital to request records.

HUC To Do—Cont'd

- Prepare a release form for the nurse to have the patient sign.
- When signed, this form may be faxed to the HIMS in the other hospital; the requested records may then be faxed to the nursing unit.
Note: If both facilities have implemented the EMR c̄ CPOE, all patient records will be available to authorized persons via computer.

Photocopying, Sending, or Faxing Medical Records

The HUC may be responsible for photocopying the records, or it may be hospital policy that they must be sent to HIMS to be photocopied. The policy for photocopying patient records should be outlined in the hospital's policies and procedures. If the EMR has been implemented, the records may be printed from the computer. The patient must sign a consent form for the records to be photocopied, printed, or faxed to another facility or to a doctor's office.

Case Management Orders

Case management is a nursing care delivery model in which a case manager (who may be a registered nurse [RN] or a social worker) coordinates the patient's care to improve quality of care, while reducing costs. The case manager interacts on a daily basis with the patient, the patient's family, health care team members, and payer representatives. Case management is not needed for every patient and is usually requested for the chronically ill, for the seriously ill or injured, and for long-term high-cost cases. The case manager acts as the patient's advocate in arranging for home health services that best suit the patient's needs, and coordinates financial coverage through private insurers such as Medicare.

The doctor may write orders requesting a case manager to access and prioritize the patient's needs, coordinate care conferences between the patient's family and physicians, identify and coordinate available resources, arrange for home care, set up admission to a long-term care facility, or plan hospice care. Most hospice care can be rendered in the patient's home, although hospice units are available in some hospital and freestanding hospice facilities.

HUC To Do

- Send the order to case management (if EMR c̄ CPOE is not implemented).
- Write the order on paper Kardex or enter into computerized Kardex (if EMR c̄ CPOE is not implemented).

Social Service Department Orders

Social Service provides much-needed information about resources available to patients and their families as they transition from the health care facility back to their home. Social workers provide many of the same services as case managers and may also work as case managers.

Social workers assist in the following:

- Patients' care-related financial matters
- Transportation home
- Meals for families staying at the hospital
- In-home meals for patients after discharge
- Teachers for long-term pediatric patients
- Living arrangements for families staying with patients
- Custodial care for patients
- Psychosocial needs of patients
- Support for abuse victims, often working with Protective Services
- Support for hospital staff after traumatic events (e.g., patient deaths, codes)

HUC To Do

Send the order to Social Services (if EMR c̄ CPOE is not implemented). Write the order on paper Kardex or enter into computerized Kardex (if EMR c̄ CPOE is not implemented).

Scheduling Orders

Frequently, while the patient is in a health care facility, the doctor may write an order to schedule the patient for various types of tests or examinations to be performed in specialized departments or outside of the health care facility. It is usually the task of the HUC to notify the department or facility that performs the test or examination and schedule a time that is convenient to the involved department and the patient and, when needed, to arrange for transportation to and from off-site testing sites. It is important to advise the patient's nurse to inform the patient and/or the patient's family of the plan and record the scheduled time on the patient's Kardex form.

Doctors' orders that may require scheduling include the following:

- Schedule pt in outpatient department for radiation therapy
- Schedule pt for psychological testing
- Schedule pt for diabetic classes
- Schedule pt for VER
- Schedule appt for dental clinic for evaluation and care

HUC To Do

- Discuss possible schedule times with the patient's nurse to avoid conflicts.
- Send or call the appropriate department to schedule tests/treatment.
- Write order with date and time of appointment on paper Kardex or enter into computerized Kardex (if EMR c̄ CPOE is not implemented).
- Notify the patient's nurse of date and time of appointment, so patient and patient's family can be notified.

Temporary Absences (passes to leave the health care facility)

Some long-term patients on rehabilitation units may be allowed to leave for 4 to 10 hours. A gradual return to society has therapeutic value for rehabilitating patients. A long-term patient may also be provided a pass to attend a wedding, funeral, graduation, or other such event.

HUC To Do

- Arrange with the pharmacy for medications the patient is taking.
- Note on the census worksheet when the patient leaves and returns.
- Cancel meals for the length of the absence.
- Cancel any hospital treatments for the length of the absence.
- Arrange for any special equipment that the patient may need.
- Provide the nurse with a temporary absence release for the patient to sign.

Other Miscellaneous Orders

Some orders do not relate to any department but are nevertheless deserving of mention. All should be Kardexed (if EMR c̄ CPOE is not implemented) in their appropriate places. Miscellaneous orders may include the following:

- Call the patient's family to come to the hospital.
  - Usually, this should be a situation in which the family would already be expecting the call.
- Diabetic nurse to do diabetic teaching with patient.
  - Many hospitals employ nurses who specialize in diabetic teaching who will work with patients in whom diabetes has been newly diagnosed. The HUC would notify the diabetic nurse of the consult.

- Have an ostomy nurse work with and train the patient in colostomy care.
  - Many hospitals employ nurses who specialize in ostomy care and teaching. The HUC would notify the ostomy nurse of the consult.
- Transfer patient to the parent teaching/transition room and teach mother to change dressings, and train in feeding tube care and feeding techniques.
  - Many pediatric hospitals and/or units have a patient room with a bed in which a parent can stay with the child. The parent, after training, will assume full care of the child while being monitored by the child's nurse. The child then may be discharged to the parent's care.
- Resp care to do preop and postop teaching.
  - This order is a request for a respiratory technician to inform a patient before their surgery what to expect and how to use an incentive spirometer. The respiratory technician would also work with the patient after surgery in assisting them to breathe and use the incentive spirometer.
- Preop teaching.
  - Preop teaching may involve breathing exercises and techniques for splinting the incision, moving in the bed, transferring to the chair, etc.
- No visitors, limited number of visitors, or have visitors speak c̄ nurse before seeing pt.
  - A sign should be posted on the patient's door to see the nurse for further explanation. The switchboard and the information desk also should be notified.
- DNR (do not resuscitate) or no code.
  - A **D**o **N**ot **R**esuscitate order may be requested by a patient upon admission. The order must be written on the patient's chart. A verbal request by a patient or a patient's family is not legal. This order is not a complete refusal of care; it simply states that a resuscitation code should not be performed in the event of cardiac or respiratory arrest. Some hospitals have DNR forms that specify the extent of resuscitative measures to be taken. The DNR order also must be written on the patient's order sheet by their doctor and, depending on the hospital's policy, must be rewritten or renewed if the patient is transferred to another unit or if there is a change in attending doctors.
- NINP (no information, no publication).
  - Various hospitals may use different abbreviations, but whatever words or abbreviations are used, this order means that the hospital staff denies that the patient is admitted when asked by visitors, either in person or by telephone. This order may be extended to include family members. Often, a code phrase or word is used for persons excluded from this restriction.

- Notify hospitalist (or resident) if systolic blood pressure (BP) >190 mm Hg.

HUC To Do

- Notify appropriate person(s) (hospital operator) or department(s).
- Make appropriate calls.
- Order appropriate supplies/equipment.
- Write order on paper Kardex or enter into computerized Kardex (if EMR c̄ CPOE is not implemented).
- Make a label for the cover of the chart if paper charts are used.

Summary

Transcribing and understanding doctors' orders is a major HUC task when paper charts are used. While you transcribe doctors' orders or monitor EMRs (when the EMR c̄ CPOE is used), you may use this Pocket Guide as a reference.

CHAPTER 9

Admission, Preoperative, Postoperative, Discharge, and Transfer Procedures and Orders

Admission Procedures

Types of Admissions

- Scheduled, or planned, admissions
- Urgent (i.e., when, in the course of a medical office visit, a doctor decides a patient needs to be admitted to a hospital)
- Direct (i.e., when a patient is seen in the hospital by his doctor for an evaluation and then is admitted)
- Elective (i.e., when a patient schedules admission for a surgical or other procedure)
- Emergency admission due to accident, sudden illness, or other medical crisis; this admission usually occurs after the patient is first seen in the hospital's emergency department or trauma center

Types of Patients

- **Inpatient**—Admitted to the hospital for longer than 24 hours
- **Observation patient**—Also called a short stay; admitted for less than 24 hours
- **Outpatient**—Receiving care in a hospital, clinic, or day surgery center but not admitted overnight or assigned to a bed. The department that is providing care processes an outpatient's orders.

Admission Order Components

Common components of admission orders include:
- Admitting diagnosis
- Diet
- Activity

- Diagnostic tests/procedures
- Medications—Usually, medications are needed for the patient's disease condition, for sleeping, and/or for pain.
- Treatment orders
- Request for old records
- Patient care category or code status—The patient care category or code status may be indicated on the patient's admission orders. The patient care category or code status refers to the patient's wishes regarding resuscitation. Code status may be written as full code, modified support, or DNR. The doctor must follow any state-specific statute and the hospital's policies and procedures when writing a DNR status.

Procedure 9-1 outlines the tasks required for admitting a patient.

✐ TAKE NOTE

Three color-coded wrist "alert" bands are now being used in many hospitals to quickly communicate a particular health care status or an "alert" that a patient may have. The different colors have specific meanings. A red wristband is used to indicate "allergy," purple indicates "do not resuscitate (DNR)," and yellow indicates a "fall risk." The words for these alerts are also written on the wristband to reduce the chance that the alert messages may be confused. The identification bracelet or wristband used is white.

Admission of a Surgical Patient

The procedure for admission of a medical or a surgical patient is the same, except that diagnostic tests ordered by the doctor are performed on surgery patients as soon as possible after their arrival to the hospital. This allows the time needed to perform diagnostic studies and have the test results added to the patient's chart before surgery is performed. An abnormal blood test result or a chest X-ray that is abnormal may require that surgery be postponed pending further evaluation.

Common Components of Orders Related Directly to Surgery

Surgeons' Orders

- **Name of surgery for surgery consent**—The consent must be signed before the patient receives any "mind-clouding" drugs. In the case of surgery that may result in sterility or loss of a limb (amputation), two permits may be required.

PROCEDURE 9–1: **Admission Procedure**

(Tasks may vary between facilities.)
When the EMR c̄ CPOE has been implemented, all tasks related to preparing a paper chart or transcribing orders would not apply.

Task	Notes
1. Greet the patient upon arrival to the nursing unit.	**1.** *Introduce yourself and give your status. Example: "I'm Ted Mart, the health unit coordinator for this unit."*
2. Inform the patient that the nurse will be notified of their arrival.	**2.** *Notify the nurse who is caring for the patient of their arrival.*
3. Notify the attending doctor and/or hospital resident or hospitalist of the patient's admission.	
4. Move the patient's name from the admission screen on the computer to the correct bed on the nursing unit.	
5. Record the patient's admission on the admission, discharge, and transfer sheet and the census board.	
6. Check the patient's signature on the admission service agreement form.	**6.** *Compare the spelling of the patient's name on the face sheet or front sheet and patient identification labels with the signature on the admission service agreement form.* *(Also check to see that the doctor's name is correct.)*
7. Complete the procedure for preparation of the paper chart.	

PROCEDURE 9–1: **Admission Procedure—Cont'd**

Task	**Notes**
a. Label all chart forms with the patient's identification labels (if paper charts are used).	
b. Fill in all needed headings (if paper charts are used).	
c. Place all forms in the chart behind the proper dividers (if paper charts are used).	
8. Label the outside of the chart (if paper charts are used).	**8.** *Identify the chart with the patient's and doctors' names and the room number.*
9. Prepare any other labels or identification cards used by the facility.	
10. Place patient identification labels in the correct place in the patient's paper chart or the correct place in the nursing unit patient label book if the EMR is used.	
11. Fill in all necessary information on the patient's Kardex form or enter it into the computer if the Kardex is computerized (if paper charts are used).	**11.** *The information is obtained from the front sheet or face sheet prepared by the admitting department and the admission nurse's notes.*
12. Place the Kardex form in the proper place in the Kardex file (if paper charts are used).	
13. Enter the appropriate required data into the computer, or scan required forms into the patient's EMR if the EMR is used.	**13.** *A patient profile requires information found on the face sheet or front sheet and the nurse's admission notes such as name, address, nearest of kin, height, weight, etc.*

(Continued)

PROCEDURE 9-1: **Admission Procedure—Cont'd**

Task	Notes
14. Record data from the admission nurse's notes onto the graphic sheet (if paper charts are used).	**14.** *The admission nurse's notes include data such as vital signs, height, and weight.*
15. Place allergy information in all designated areas, or write "NKA" (if paper charts are used).	**15.** *Allergy information (information obtained from the patient about any sensitivity to medication, food, or other substance) is usually placed on the front of the patient's chart, Kardex form, and medication record. Allergy information is obtained from the admission nurse's notes. Writing "NKA" indicates to staff that the allergy information has been checked.*
16. Prepare an allergy bracelet with allergies written on it to be placed on the patient's wrist if necessary.	
17. Note code status on the front of the chart if necessary (if paper charts are used).	
18. Place a label or piece of red tape stating "name alert" on the spine of the chart if a patient with the same or a similar name is on the unit (if paper charts are used).	
19. Transcribe the admission orders according to hospital policy (if paper charts are used).	

- **Enemas**—The order for an enema depends on the type of surgery. For surgeries within the abdominal cavity, all wastes must be removed from the intestines. This allows the surgeon more room for exploration and a clear field of vision, and it decreases the danger of contamination and infection.
- **Shaves, scrubs, or showers**—The site of the surgical incision must be prepared. The surgeon also may require a special scrub at the surgical site. In some facilities, operating room staff members may do shaves and scrubs. Often, the doctor writes an order for the patient to take a shower before surgery using an antibacterial soap such as Hibiclens.
- **Name of anesthesiologist or anesthesiology group**—It is necessary to know the anesthesiologist's name or specific anesthesiology group in the event that preoperative medication orders are not received. The HUC may then call the anesthesiologist, group, or person responsible for writing the **preoperative orders**. (In hospitals where nurse anesthetists administer the anesthesia, the surgeon may write the preoperative anesthesia orders.)
- **Miscellaneous orders**—Other orders may include Ted hose, additional diagnostic studies, blood components to be given during surgery, or intravenous preparations to be started before surgery. Treatments and additional medications also may be ordered.

Anesthesiologists' Orders

- **Diet**—When surgery is to be performed during the morning hours, the patient is usually NPO (nothing by mouth) at midnight. For a patient who is having late afternoon surgery, an order may be written for a clear liquid breakfast at 0600 and then NPO.
- **Preoperative medications**—The anesthesiologist or the surgeon usually writes an order for preoperative medication for the patient who is scheduled for surgery.

Procedure 9-2 outlines the tasks required for transcribing preoperative orders.

Surgical Procedure Abbreviations That May Be Included in Doctors' Orders*

A & A	arthroscopy and arthrotomy
AKA	above the knee amputation
A & P repair	anterior and posterior colporrhaphy
A & P resection	abdominoperineal resection
AV fistula	arteriovenous fistula
AVR	aortic valve replacement
AV shunt	atrial/ventricular shunt
BKA	below the knee amputation
BSO	bilateral salpingo-oophorectomy

*These abbreviations would have to be spelled out on the surgery consent form. Abbreviations are not legal on a consent form.

Surgical Procedure Abbreviations That May Be Included in Doctors' Orders*—Cont'd

Bx	biopsy
CABG	coronary artery bypass graft
CR	closed reduction
D & C	dilation and curettage
DSA	diagnostic surgical arthroscopy
ECCE	extracapsular cataract extraction
EHL	electrohydraulic lithotripsy
ESWL	extracorporeal shock wave lithotripsy
EUA	examination under anesthesia
Exp Lap	exploratory laparotomy
FESS	fiberoptic endoscopic sinus surgery
FTSG	full-thickness skin graft
ICBG	iliac crest bone graft
LEEP	loop electrosurgical excision procedure
MMK	Marshall Marchetti Krantz
MMX	medial meniscectomy
MUA	manipulation under anesthesia
ORIF	open reduction, internal fixation
PEG	percutaneous endoscopic gastrostomy
PTCA	percutaneous transluminal coronary angioplasty
STSG	split-thickness skin graft
T & A	tonsillectomy and adenoidectomy
TAH	total abdominal hysterectomy
THA	total hip arthroscopy
THR	total hip replacement
TKA	total knee arthroscopy
TKR	total knee replacement
TURB	transurethral resection of the bladder
TURBN	transurethral resection of the bladder neck
TURP	transurethral resection of the prostate
TVH	total vaginal hysterectomy
TVR	tricuspid valve replacement
UPPP	uvulopalatopharyngoplasty
VATS	video-assisted thoracic surgery
	video-assisted thoracoscopic surgery

These abbreviations would have to be spelled out on the surgery consent form. Abbreviations are not legal on a consent form.

Postoperative orders that relate to the patient's treatment after surgery usually contain the following components:

- **Diet**—The patient may remain NPO or may be given "sips and chips." The diet then is increased as tolerated.
- **I & O**—The patient's intake and output is closely watched for 24 to 48 hours.

PROCEDURE 9-2: **Preoperative Procedure**

(Tasks may vary between facilities.)
When the EMR c̄ CPOE has been implemented, all tasks related to preparing a paper chart or transcribing orders would not apply.

Task	Notes
1. Label surgery forms with the patient's identification labels and place them within the patient's paper chart (if paper charts are used).	**1.** *Surgery forms include nurse's preoperative checklist, anesthesiologist's record, operating room record, recovery room record, etc. Forms vary among hospitals.*
2. Check the patient's chart for history and physical report (if paper charts are used).	**2.** *If a history and physical report is not found on the chart, call the health information management services/department (HIMS) to check whether it has been dictated. Notify the patient's nurse and doctor if the report is not located.*
3. Check the patient's paper or electronic chart for the following signed consent forms:	**3.** *Check consent forms for the patient's and witness's signatures and for correct spelling of the surgical procedure.*
a. Surgical consent	
b. Blood transfusion consent or refusal form	
c. Admission service agreement	
4. Check the patient's paper chart for any previously ordered diagnostic studies such as laboratory tests, X-rays, and so forth. If the EMR is used, check the computer screen for any HUC tasks.	**4.** *If diagnostic test results are not included on the patient's chart, locate results on the computer, print, and place them in the patient's chart. If you are unable to locate results, notify the patient's nurse.*

(Continued)

PROCEDURE 9–2: **Preoperative Procedure—Cont'd**

Task	Notes
5. Chart the patient's latest vital signs (if paper charts are used).	
6. File the current medication administration record in the patient's chart (if paper charts are used).	
7. Print at least five face sheets to place in the paper chart. If the EMR is used, maintain five face sheets in a notebook to provide to consulting doctors and other health care providers as requested.	**7.** *Face sheets are removed and used by doctors and other health care providers to bill patients.*
8. Place at least three sheets of patient identification labels in the patient's paper chart. If the EMR is used, maintain three sheets of labels in a notebook to label specimens as necessary.	**8.** *Patient identification labels are used to label specimens.*
9. Notify appropriate nursing personnel when surgery calls for the patient.	**9.** *Usually, surgery personnel will call before they send transport, to verify that the patient is prepared to be picked up.*

- **IV fluids**—For most surgery patients, at least one bag of intravenous fluids is ordered after surgery.
- **Vital signs (VS)**—The patient's vital signs are monitored carefully after surgery, usually every 4 hours for 24 to 48 hours.
- **Catheters, tubes, and drains**—Postoperative patients may have a retention (indwelling) urinary catheter. Other orders may pertain to intermittent catheterization of the patient, as necessary. Some patients may require suctioning when nasogastric or other tubes are in place.
- **Activity**—Activity after surgery may consist of only bed rest, and this may be increased as the patient continues to recuperate.

- **Positioning**—Some surgeons require that the patient's position be changed frequently. Elevation of the bed also may be very important.
- **Observation of the operative site**—It is imperative that the sites of the operation or the bandages be observed closely for bleeding, excessive drainage, redness, and swelling.
- **Medications**—Medications to relieve pain (narcotics) and nausea and vomiting (antiemetics) and to help the patient sleep or rest (hypnotics) may be prescribed for a period after surgery. Other medications are ordered as needed. Procedure 9-3 outlines the tasks required for transcribing postoperative orders.

PROCEDURE 9-3: **Postoperative Procedure**

(Tasks may vary between facilities.)
When the EMR c̄ CPOE has been implemented, all tasks related to transcribing orders would not apply.

Task	Notes
1. Inform the patient's nurse of the patient's arrival to the postanesthesia care unit (PACU) as soon as possible.	*1. PACU personnel usually notify the unit when the patient arrives from the operating room. The nurse then may plan and may be prepared for the patient's return to the unit.*
2. Inform the patient's nurse of the expected arrival of the patient from the recovery room.	*2. PACU personnel will notify the nursing unit before they return the patient to their room and will give a report of the patient's condition to the appropriate nurse.*
3. Place all operating records behind the proper divider in patient's chart.	*3. Check consent forms for the patient's and witness's signatures and for correct spelling of the surgical procedure.*
4. Write date of surgery and surgical procedure in the designated place on patient's Kardex form or in computer.	
5. Write in date of surgery on patient's graphic sheet.	

(Continued)

PROCEDURE 9-3: **Postoperative Procedure—Cont'd**	

Task	Notes
6. Transcribe doctors' postoperative orders. Notify nurse caring for patient of stat doctors' orders.	**6.** *All preoperative orders are automatically discontinued postoperatively. The HUC usually starts a new Kardex form for the patient.*

Five types of discharges may occur:
1. Discharge home
2. Discharge to another facility
3. Discharge home with assistance
4. Discharge against medical advice (AMA)
5. Expiration (death)

All discharges require a doctor's order. When a patient insists on leaving against medical advice, the doctor usually writes a discharge order with documentation that the patient is leaving against medical advice. It is important for staff members to read a discharge order carefully before a patient leaves the unit. The doctor may write "discharge after chest X-ray" or may write other directions and/or may leave a prescription on the chart to give to the patient. Procedure 9-4 outlines the tasks required for transcribing routine discharge orders.

Patients may be discharged to an assisted living facility, a nursing care home, or an extended care facility/skilled nursing facility (ECF/SNF). Usually, the hospital case manager or social service worker makes the arrangements for long-term care. The discharge of a patient to another facility is the same as a routine discharge with additional steps. Procedure 9-5 outlines the tasks required for transcribing discharge to another facility orders.

Many patients need care or assistance at home as part of their recovery process. Additional steps are required when a patient needs home health care. The hospital case manager or social service worker arranges home health care and home health equipment. Procedure 9-6 outlines the tasks required for transcribing discharge home with assistance orders.

PROCEDURE 9–4: **Routine Discharge Procedure**

Task	Notes
1. Read the entire order when you transcribe the discharge order.	**1.** *The order may be written on the doctors' order sheet on the day before or on the day of the expected discharge. Read the order carefully. Sometimes, the doctor will write "disch c̄ chest X-ray" or other diagnostic test. Check for any Rx that may have been left in the chart by the doctor.*
2. Notify the discharged patient's nurse.	**2.** *The patient's nurse will provide the patient with discharge instructions. When the EMR c̄ CPOE is implemented, the HUC may print discharge instructions from the computer for the patient. The HUC also may print out medication information sheets for medications the patient will be taking after discharge.*
3. Enter "pending discharge" with expected departure time into computer.	**3.** *Notification may be made by telephone or by computer. Entering "pending discharge" with expected departure time notifies the business department to prepare the patient's bill. Some patients may be required to stop at the business office before leaving the hospital. A "pending discharge" notification also alerts the admitting department that patients waiting to be admitted may be placed into a room slot. Holding notification of discharge could delay another patient's admission and the start of treatment.*

(Continued)

PROCEDURE 9–4: **Routine Discharge Procedure—Cont'd**

Task

4. Explain the discharge procedure to the patient and/or the patient's relatives.

5. Notify other departments that may be giving the patient daily treatments.

6. Communicate the patient's discharge to the Nutritional Care department by computer.

7. Arrange for any appointments requested by the doctor.

8. Arrange transportation if needed.

9. Prepare credit slips for medications returned to the pharmacy or equipment and supplies to the CSD.

Notes

4. *An explanation of the discharge procedure may also be given by the nurse; however, many patients come to the nurses' station to ask the HUC for the explanation.*

5. *Departments such as Physical Therapy and Cardiopulmonary (Respiratory Care) may have to be notified. This information may be communicated by telephone or by computer.*

6. *If the patient is not planning to leave the hospital during regular discharge hours (usually before lunch), type in the expected departure time.*

7. *Write out the appointment date and time on a piece of paper, and give it to the patient's nurse. The appointment date and time may then be written on or typed into the discharge instruction sheet.*

8. *Patients who do not have family or friends available to provide transportation may have to have a taxi called. Many hospitals provide taxi vouchers for patients.*

9. *Supplies specifically ordered for the patient from the CSD but not used by the patient must be returned to the CSD with a credit slip.*

PROCEDURE 9–4: **Routine Discharge Procedure—Cont'd**

Task	Notes
10. Notify nursing personnel or transportation service to transport the patient to the discharge area when the patient is ready to leave.	**10.** *Never allow patients to go to the discharge area without escort from hospital staff. Also, the patient should be transported via a wheelchair.*
11. Write the patient's name on the admission, discharge, and transfer sheets.	
12. Delete the patient's name from the unit census board and the temperature, pulse, and respiration (TPR) sheets.	**12.** *Draw a line through the patient's name on the TPR sheet, and erase their name on the census board (applicable when paper charts are used).*
13. Notify Environmental Services to clean the discharged patient's room.	**13.** *Notification may be made by telephone, by computer, or by telling Environmental Services personnel on the unit.*
14. Prepare the patient's paper chart for HIMS.	**14.** *Many hospitals issue a discharge checklist to prepare the chart for HIMS (applicable when paper charts are used).*
a. Check the summary/ diagnosis-related group (DRG) worksheet for the doctor's summation and the patient's final diagnosis. It is important to have this information upon patient discharge so that coding of DRGs may be placed on the chart by HIMS personnel.	*Applicable when paper charts are used.*
b. Check for correct patient identification labels on the chart forms.	*Applicable when paper charts are used.*

(Continued)

PROCEDURE 9-4: **Routine Discharge Procedure—Cont'd**

Task	Notes
c. Shred all chart forms labeled with no documentation on them.	*Applicable when paper charts are used.*
d. Check for old records or split records, and send with the chart to HIMS.	
e. Arrange the chart forms in discharge sequence according to your hospital policy.	
f. Send the chart of the discharged patient to HIMS along with any old records of the patient. Paper charts of discharged patients must be sent to HIMS on the day of discharge.	*After the patient's paper chart has been sent to HIMS, nurses, doctors, residents, and other health care providers will have to go there to complete charting or to sign forms if necessary.*

PROCEDURE 9-5: **Additional Steps to Discharge Patient to Another Facility**

Task	Notes
1. Notify case management or social service of doctors' orders to discharge to another facility.	
2. Transportation usually will be arranged by the case manager or social worker.	**2.** *A patient who is confined to bed or who has other special medical needs may require an ambulance when requested.*
3. Complete a continuing care form or transfer form.	**3.** *A continuing care form requires some information that the HUC may fill in from the face sheet. The nurse and the doctor complete specific sections of the form.*

PROCEDURE 9–5: **Additional Steps to Discharge Patient to Another Facility—Cont'd**

Task	Notes
4. Photocopy or print from the computer the patient chart forms, as indicated in the doctors' orders.	**4.** *The requirement of forms will vary from facility to facility. The patient's doctor will write an order indicating specific forms to be photocopied or printed from the computer. It is also necessary to check hospital policy to determine who is responsible for making photocopies or for printing them from the computer (HUC or HIMS). Once copies have been made, it is important that paper originals be placed back in the chart in proper sequence.*
5. Distribute the continuing care form and copies as required.	**5.** *Photocopies and a copy of the continuing care form are placed in a sealed envelope to be given to the ambulance driver or a family member. This person delivers the envelope to the nurse at the nursing care facility.*
6. Now, perform all routine steps as shown in Procedure 9–4.	

PROCEDURE 9–6: Additional Steps for Discharge Home With Assistance

Task	Notes
1. Notify case management or social service of the doctor's order.	1. *Responsible personnel to be notified will vary depending on patient type.*
2. Prepare the continuing care form.	2. *The HUC should complete the personal information section.*
3. Obtain the release of information signature from the patient.	
4. Photocopy or print forms as indicated in the doctors' order.	
5. Distribute the continuing care form and copies as required.	
6. Now, perform routine discharge steps.	

Discharge Against Medical Advice

A patient may appear at the nurses' station and announce that they are leaving the hospital. The HUC should ask the patient to be seated until their nurse is advised. The hospitalist, resident, or admitting doctor may be called to speak with the patient. The patient may be advised that their insurance will not cover the hospital bill if they leave against medical advice. Everything possible is done to encourage the patient to remain in the hospital until the treatment is completed. However, if the patient does not pose a threat to self or others, they cannot be restrained from leaving, and usually the admitting doctor, resident, or hospitalist will write a discharge order with the documentation that the patient is leaving against medical advice.

✐ TAKE NOTE

A patient may be restrained from leaving the hospital if two doctors certify that the patient poses a threat to self or others.

In the event that the patient is not convinced to stay, a release form is prepared. The form is signed by the patient or their representative, and the signing is witnessed by an appropriate member of the hospital staff. The patient then is permitted to leave the hospital, and the discharge procedure is the same as for a routine discharge.

Discharge of the Deceased Patient

Patient Deaths

The HUC may be requested to call a member of the clergy from a specific religion to speak with the patient or to perform final rites. Most facilities have a list of representatives from various denominations and nondenominational groups to assist patients and families, and many hospitals may employ a chaplain to meet religious needs. A notation should be made on the patient's Kardex form of any final rites that have been performed. It is important to remind clergy that a lighted candle cannot be used when oxygen is in use in the patient's room.

Certification of Death

The hospitalist, resident, or doctor must be notified to pronounce the patient dead. The patient is examined for any signs of life. If none can be detected, the patient is pronounced dead and the official time is recorded on the doctors' progress notes. The patient's doctor must complete a death certificate, and a report of the death must be filed with the Bureau of Vital Statistics.

Release of Remains

The patient's family or guardian must indicate the funeral home to which the body will be released. Usually, the family must sign a form before the patient can be released to the funeral home. The nursing staff or the HUC (when requested to do so) may notify the funeral home of the expiration. The HUC may be asked to call the hospital morgue personnel to take the deceased patient to the morgue. The funeral home personnel may pick up the patient from the unit or the hospital morgue. A hospital security officer may need to accompany the funeral home personnel.

Organ Donation

Many patients indicate their wishes for organ donation before the time of their death. A patient may designate specific organs (e.g., cornea only) or any needed organs or tissues. Because of state laws, nursing staff may be required to ask the family about organ donation and must check the hospital's policies regarding organ donation. Additional consent forms are necessary for the harvesting of an organ (organ procurement).

Autopsy or Postmortem Examination

The family may ask that an autopsy be done, or the doctor may request it. Before an autopsy can be performed, however, the family must grant permission. A consent for autopsy form must be signed by the next of kin.

Coroner's Cases

A coroner's case is one in which the patient's death is due to sudden, violent, or unexplained circumstances such as an accident, a poisoning, or a gunshot wound. Deaths that occur less than 24 hours after hospitalization also may be called *coroner's cases.* State, county, and local governments have regulations that define a coroner's case in their particular locality. The law gives the coroner permission to study the body by dissection to determine whether there is evidence of foul play. A consent form signed by the nearest of kin is not required or necessary when a death is ruled a coroner's case. See Procedure 9-7 for tasks related to the death of a patient, which may be performed by the HUC.

PROCEDURE 9-7: **Postmortem Procedure**

Task	Notes
1. Contact the attending doctor, hospitalist, or resident when asked by the nurse to do so, to verify the patient's death.	
2. Notify the hospital operator of the patient's death.	
3. Prepare any needed forms.	**3.** *Forms may consist of release of remains/request for autopsy and/or consent for donation of body organs. Some hospitals use a postmortem checklist to ascertain that all postmortem tasks have been completed.*

PROCEDURE 9–7: **Postmortem Procedure—Cont'd**

Task	Notes
4. Notify the mortuary as requested by the family.	**4.** *If the family is not familiar with mortuaries in the area, a list is usually available from the hospital telephone switchboard operator. Nursing office personnel may notify the funeral home.*
5. Check the chart or ask the patient's nurse to determine whether the body is to be taken to the morgue or is to remain there until the mortician arrives.	**5.** *Sometimes, the family will request that the patient remain in the hospital room so additional family members may see them.*
6. The nurse will gather the clothing of the deceased patient and will place it in a patient belongings bag to be labeled with the patient's name, room number, and date.	**6.** *Clothing is given to the family or to the mortician.*
7. Obtain the mortuary book from the nursing office, or have the mortuary form prepared when the mortician arrives.	**7.** *The mortician who claims the body must complete forms to show that they claimed the body, clothing, and any valuables.*
8. Notify all doctors who were involved with the patient's care.	
9. Now, perform routine discharge steps as shown in Procedure 9–4.	

Transfer of a Patient

The duties performed in a series of tasks allow for an orderly transfer of the patient from one area to another. Procedure 9-8 lists tasks to perform when receiving a transferred patient. Transfer may occur from one unit of the hospital to another (Procedure 9-9), or it may involve movement from one room to another on the same nursing unit (Procedure 9-10).

PROCEDURE 9–8: **Procedure for a Receiving a Transferred Patient**

Task	Notes
1. Notify the nurse who is caring for the patient of the expected arrival of the transferred patient.	
2. Introduce yourself to the transferred patient upon arrival to the unit.	
3. Notify the nurse who is caring for the patient of the transferred patient's arrival.	
4. Place the patient's paper chart in the correct slot in the chart holder, print the corrected patient ID labels, and label the patient's chart (if paper charts are used).	**4.** *Provide an empty chart to the unit from which the patient was transferred.*
5. Place the Kardex form in its proper place (if paper charts are used).	
6. Record the receiving of the transfer patient on the unit admission, discharge, and transfer sheets, and write the patient's name on the census board.	
7. Place the patient's name on the temperature, pulse, and respirations (TPR) sheet (if paper charts are used), and notify the Nutritional Care department of the patient's transfer.	
8. Move the patient's name from the unit the patient came from and place it in the correct bed on the computer census screen.	

PROCEDURE 9–8: **Procedure for a Receiving a Transferred Patient—Cont'd**

Task	Notes
9. Transcribe any new doctors' orders (if paper charts are used).	**9.** *When the patient is transferred from the intensive care unit (ICU) to a regular unit, or from a regular unit to the ICU, the doctor must write new orders. Previous ICU orders are no longer valid.*

PROCEDURE 9–9: **Procedure for Transfer From One Unit to Another**

Task	Notes
1. Transcribe the order for transfer.	**1.** *The transfer order may be handwritten when paper charts are used or may be indicated by an icon on the computer census screen next to the appropriate patient's name when the EMR is used.*
2. Notify the nurse who is caring for the patient of the transfer order.	
3. Notify the Admitting department of the transfer order to obtain a new room assignment.	
4. Communicate new unit and room assignment to the nurse who is caring for the patient.	
5. Notify the receiving unit of the transfer by telephone or by computer.	
6. Record the transfer on a unit admission, discharge, and transfer sheet.	

(Continued)

PROCEDURE 9–9: **Procedure for Transfer From One Unit to Another—Cont'd**

Task	Notes
7. Send all thinned records, old records (if paper charts are used), and X-rays with the patient to the receiving unit.	
8. Send the patient's chart, Kardex form, and current medication administration record (MAR) with the patient to the receiving unit (if paper charts are used).	8. *An empty chart will be given in exchange for the patient's chart by the receiving unit (if paper charts are used).*
9. Usually, the nurse puts medications in a bag to be sent with the paper chart.	
10. Erase the patient's name from the census board.	
11. Notify all departments that perform regularly scheduled treatments on the patient.	
12. Indicate the transfer on the diet sheet or in the computer and on the temperature, pulse, and respirations (TPR) sheet (if paper charts are used).	
13. Notify Environmental Services to clean the room.	13. *Environmental Services may be notified by telephone, by computer, or in person.*
14. Notify the attending doctor and all other doctors involved in the patient's care, as well as the information desk, of the transfer.	

PROCEDURE 9-10: **Procedure to Transfer to Another Room on the Same Unit**

Task	Notes
1. Transcribe the order for transfer.	**1.** *The transfer order may be handwritten when paper charts are used or may be indicated by icon on computer census screen next to the appropriate patient's name when the EMR is used.*
2. Notify the nurse who is caring for the patient of the request for transfer.	
3. Place the patient's chart in the correct slot in the chart rack after you have corrected labels on the patient's chart and have replaced patient ID labels with corrected labels (if paper charts are used).	
4. Place the Kardex form in its new place in the Kardex form file (if paper charts are used).	
5. Move the patient's name to the correct bed on the computer census screen. Send the change to the Nutritional Care department and change the room number on the temperature, pulse, and respirations (TPR) sheet (if paper charts are used).	
6. Record the transfer on the unit admission, discharge, and transfer sheet.	
7. Notify Environmental Services that the patient's room must be cleaned.	**7.** *Environmental Services may be notified by telephone, by computer, or in person.*
8. Notify the switchboard information center of the change.	

Summary

The tasks of the HUC in admission, preoperative, postoperative, discharge, and transfer procedures are many when the paper chart is used. Some of these tasks remain the same and additional tasks may be required when the EMR is implemented. If the HUC learns these procedures in a particular order and does not deviate from them, they will always be performed thoroughly and completely.

Abbreviations

The following is a list of alphabetized abbreviations that are used frequently in doctors' orders. Most of the abbreviations related to specific departments, such as laboratory and diagnostic imaging, are not included here. For those, please refer to the chapters that discuss those departments.

Abbreviation	Meaning
>	greater than
<	less than
↑	increase or above
/	per or by
Δ	change
@	at
↓	decrease or below
°	degree or hour
A	apical
AA	active assisted
A&A	arthroscopy and arthrotomy
ā	before
āā	of each
AAROM	active-assistive range of motion
Ab	antibody
abd	abdominal
ABG	arterial blood gas
ABR	absolute bed rest
ac	before meals
ACL	anterior cruciate ligament repair
ADA	American Diabetic Association
ADE	adverse drug event
ADH	antidiuretic hormone (chemistry)
ADL	activity(ies) of daily living

Abbreviation	Meaning
ad lib	as desired
A-drive	floppy drive
ADS	adult distress syndrome
ADT Log Book	a book used to record all admissions, discharges, and transfers on a nursing unit
ADT Sheet	a form used to record admissions, discharges, and transfers on a nursing unit for each day
AE	antiembolism
AFB	acid-fast bacillus
Ag	antigen
AHA	American Heart Association
AIDS	acquired immunodeficiency syndrome
AKA	above the knee amputation
ALP or alk phos	alkaline phosphatase (chemistry)
A.M.	morning
AMA	against medical advice
amb	ambulate
AMO	against medical orders
amp	ampule
ANA	American Nurses Association; antinuclear antibody (serology)
ANCC	American Nurses Credentialing Center
A&O	alert and oriented
AP	anteroposterior
A&P repair	anterior and posterior colporrhaphy
A&P resection	abdominoperineal resection
appt	appointment
APS	Adult Protective Services
ARC	AIDS-related complex
ARDS	acute (adult) respiratory distress syndrome
AROM	active range of motion
ASA	acetylsalicylic acid (aspirin)
ASAP	as soon as possible
as tol	as tolerated
AV fistula	arteriovenous fistula
AV shunt	atrial/ventricular shunt
ax	axillary
BAER or AER	brainstem auditory response
BC	blood culture
BCOC	bowel care of choice
BE	barium enema
BIBA	brought in by ambulance
bid	twice a day
bili	bilirubin
BiPap	bilevel positive airway pressure

Abbreviation	Meaning
BiW, biw	twice a week
BKA	below the knee amputation
B/L	bilateral
BLE	both lower extremities
BM	bowel movement
BMI	body mass index
BMP	basic metabolic panel
BNP	brain natriuretic peptide
BP	blood pressure
BR	bed rest
BRP	bathroom privileges
BS	blood sugar
BSC	bedside commode
BUE	both upper extremities
BUN	blood urea nitrogen
Bx	biopsy
$\bar{c}$	with
C	Celsius
Ca	cancer
Ca or Ca$^+$	calcium
CABG	coronary artery bypass graft
CAD	coronary artery disease
cal	calorie
cap	capsule
CAT	computed axial tomography
cath	catheterize
CBC	complete blood cell count
CBG	capillary blood gas
CBI	continuous bladder irrigation
CBR	continuous bed rest
cc or cm^3	cubic centimeter
CC, creat cl, or cr cl	creatinine clearance (chemistry)
CCM	certified case manager
CCU	coronary care unit
CDC	Centers for Disease Control and Prevention
C-drive	hard drive stored inside the computer
CDSS	clinical decision support system/s
CE	covered entities
CEA	carcinoembryonic antigen (special chemistry)
CEO	chief executive officer
CFO	chief financial officer
CHF	congestive heart failure
CHO	carbohydrate
chol	cholesterol
CHUC	certified health unit coordinator

Abbreviation	Meaning
CI	clinical indication
Cl	chloride (chemistry)
cl	clear
cm	centimeter
CMP	comprehensive metabolic panel
CMS	circulation, motion, sensation
CMT	cardiac monitor technician
CMV	cytomegalovirus
CNA	certified nursing assistant
c/o	complained of
CO_2	carbon dioxide
COA or C of A	condition of admission
comp or cmpd	compound
con't	continue
COO	chief operating officer
COPD	chronic obstructive pulmonary disease
COW	computer on wheels
CP	cold pack
CPAP	continuous positive airway pressure
CPK or CK	creatine phosphokinase or creatine kinase (chemistry)
CPM	continuous passive motion
CPOE	computer physician order entry
CPR	cardiopulmonary resuscitation
CPS	Child Protective Services
CPT	chest physical therapy
CPU	central processing unit
CPZ	Compazine
CQI	continuous quality improvement
C&S	culture and sensitivity
CSF	cerebrospinal fluid
CT	computed tomography
CVA	cerebrovascular accident
CVC	central venous catheter
CVICU	cardiovascular intensive critical care unit
CVP	central venous pressure
Cx	culture
CXR	chest X-ray
D or E drive	drive/s to read CDs or DVDs
DAT	diet as tolerated; direct antiglobulin test
D/C or DC	discontinue
	discharge
Diff	differential
Dig	digoxin
Disch	discharge

Abbreviation	Meaning
D/LR	dextrose in lactated Ringer's solution
DME	durable medical equipment
DMS	document management system
DNR	do not resuscitate
D/NS	dextrose in normal saline
DO	doctor of osteopathy
DOA	dead on arrival
DPI	dry powder inhaler
dr or $\mathfrak{z}$	dram
DRG	diagnosis-related group
D/RL	dextrose in Ringer's lactate
DSA	digital subtraction angiography
DSS	dioctyl sodium sulfosuccinate (Colace)
DSU	day surgery unit
D/W	dextrose in water
DW	distilled water
D_5W	5% dextrose in water
$D_{10}W$	10% dextrose in water
Dx	diagnosis
EBV	Epstein-Barr virus
EC	enteric coated
ECF	extended care facility
ECG or EKG	electrocardiogram
ED	emergency department
EEG	electroencephalogram
EGD	esophagogastroduodenoscopy
elix	elixir
EMG	electromyogram
EMR/EHR	electronic medical (health) record
ENG	electronystagmography
EPC	electronic pain control
EPHI	electronic protected health information
EPS	electrophysiologic study
ER	emergency room
ERCP	endoscopic retrograde cholangiopancreatography
ES	electrical stimulation
ESR	erythrocyte sedimentation rate
ESRD	end-stage renal disease
ET	endotracheal tube
ETS	elevated toilet seat
F	Fahrenheit
FBS	fasting blood sugar
Fe	iron
FF	force fluids

Abbreviation	Meaning
FFP	fresh frozen plasma
fib	fibrinogen
FPG	fasting plasma glucose (chemistry)
FS	full strength
	frozen section
5-FU	5-fluorouracil
F/U	follow-up
FWB	full weight bearing
FWW	front wheel walker
Fx, fx	fracture
G, gm, g	gram
GB	gallbladder
GI	gastrointestinal
gluc	glucose
gr	grain
GTT	glucose tolerance test
gtt(s)	drop(s)
Gyn	gynecology
h, hr, hrs	hour/s
h or (H)	hypodermic
HA	heated aerosol
H/A	headache
HBOT	hyperbaric O_2 therapy
HB_sAg	hepatitis B surface antigen
HBV	hepatitis B virus
hCG	human chorionic gonadotropin
hct	hematocrit
HCTZ	hydrochlorothiazide
HCV	hepatitis C virus
HD	hemodialysis
HDL	high-density lipoprotein
hgb	hemoglobin
H&H	hemoglobin and hematocrit
HIMS	health information management system
HIPAA	Health Insurance Portability and Accountability Act
HIV	human immunodeficiency virus
HIVB24Ag	human immunodeficiency virus antigen screen (serology)
HL or hep-lock	heparin lock
HMO	health maintenance organization
HNP	herniated nucleus pulposus
HO	house officer
h/o	history of
H_2O	water

Abbreviation	Meaning
H₂O₂	hydrogen peroxide
HOB	head of bed
H&P	history and physical
HP	hot pack
hs	bedtime
HSV	herpes simplex virus
HUC	health unit coordinator
	health unit clerk
HUS	health unit secretary
Hx	history
ICD	implantable cardioverter-defibrillator
	International Classification of Diseases
ICU	intensive care unit
ID labels	identification labels
IIHI	individually identifiable health information
IM	intramuscular
I&O	intake and output
IPG	impedance plethysmography
IPPB	intermittent positive-pressure breathing
irrig	irrigate
IS	incentive spirometry
ISOM	isometric
IV	intravenous
IVDU	intravenous drug user
IVF	intravenous fluids
IVP	intravenous pyelogram
IVPB	intravenous piggyback
IVU	intravenous urogram
K	potassium
KCl	potassium chloride
kg	kilogram
KO	keep open
KUB	kidneys, ureters, and bladder
L	liter
lat	lateral
lb, #	pound(s)
L&D	labor and delivery
LDL	low-density lipoprotein
LE	lower extremity
liq	liquid
LLE	left lower extremity
LLL	left lower lobe
LLQ	left lower quadrant
L/min	liters per minute

Abbreviation	Meaning
LOC	laxative of choice
	leave on chart
	level of consciousness
	loss of consciousness
LP	lumbar puncture
LPN	licensed practical nurse
LR	lactated Ringer's solution
L&S	liver and spleen
LS	lumbosacral
Lt or Ⓛ	left
LTC	long-term care
LUE	left upper extremity
LUL	left upper lobe
LUQ	left upper quadrant
lytes or e-lytes	electrolytes
MAR	medication administration record
MD	doctor of medicine
MDI	metered-dose inhaler
Med	medical
mEq	milliequivalent
mets	metastasis
μg, mcg	microgram
mg	milligram
Mg or Mg⁺	magnesium
MgSO	magnesium sulfate
MI	myocardial infarction
MICU	medical intensive care unit
min	minute
mL	milliliter
MN	midnight
MOM	Milk of Magnesia
MR	may repeat
MRI	magnetic resonance imaging
MRSA	methicillin-resistant *Staphylococcus aureus*
MSO$_4$ or MS	morphine sulfate
MSSU	medical short-stay unit
Na or Na⁺	sodium
NAHUC	National Association of Health Unit Coordinators
NAS	no added salt
NCS	nerve conduction study
nec	necessary
Neuro	neurology
NG	nasogastric
NICU	neonatal intensive care unit

Abbreviation	Meaning
NINP	no information, no publication
NKA	no known allergies
NKDA	no known drug allergies
NKFA	no known food allergies
NKMA	no known medication allergies
noc	night
non rep	do not repeat
NP	nasopharynx
NPO	nothing by mouth
NS	normal saline
NSA	no salt added
NTG	nitroglycerin
N/V	nausea and vomiting
NVS or neuro ✓s	neurologic vital signs or checks
NWB	non–weight bearing
O_2	oxygen
OB	obstetrics
OBS	observation
OCG	oral cholecystogram
OD	right eye
OOB	out of bed
O&P	ova and parasites
OPS	outpatient surgery
OR	operating room
ORE	oil-retention enema
ORIF	open reduction, internal fixation
Ortho	orthopedics
OS	left eye
OSA	obstructive sleep apnea
OSHA	Occupational Safety and Health Administration
OSMO	osmolality
OT	occupational therapy
OTC	over-the-counter
OU	both eyes
oz	ounce
p̄	after
P	pulse
PA	posteroanterior
PACS	Picture Archiving and Communication Systems
PACU	postanesthesia care unit
PAP	prostatic acid phosphatase
PAS	pulsatile antiembolism stockings
PBZ	pyribenzamine
PC	personal computer; packed cell
pc	after meals

Abbreviation	Meaning
PCA	patient-controlled analgesia
PCN	penicillin
PCP	primary care physician
PCT	patient care technician
PCV	packed-cell volume (hematology; same as hematocrit)
PCXR	portable chest X-ray
PD	peritoneal dialysis
PDPV	postural drainage, percussion, and vibration
PDR	*Physicians' Desk Reference*
Peds	pediatrics
PEEP	positive end-expiratory pressure
PEG	percutaneous endoscopic gastrostomy
PEP	positive expiratory pressure
PET	positron emission tomography
pH	hydrogen ion concentration (acidity)
PHI	protected health information reference
PICC	peripherally inserted central catheter
PICU	pediatric intensive care unit
PID	pelvic inflammatory disease
PKU	phenylketonuria (chemistry)
P.M.	evening, night
PO	by mouth, or postoperative
PO_4 or phos	phosphate or phosphorus (chemistry)
POCT or PCT	point-of-care testing performed on the nursing unit
Postop, postop	after surgery
PP	postpartum
pp	postprandial (after meals)
P&PD	percussion and postural drainage
PPE	personal protective equipment
PPO	preferred provider organization
pr	per rectum
Preop, preop	before surgery
prn	whenever necessary
PROM	passive range of motion
PSA	patient support associate
	prostate-specific antigen
Psych	psychiatry
PT	physical therapy; prothrombin time
Pt	patient
PTA	physical therapy assistant
PTCA	percutaneous transluminal coronary angioplasty
PTHC or PTC	percutaneous transhepatic cholangiography

Abbreviation	Meaning
PTT or APTT	partial thromboplastin time or activated partial thromboplastin time
PWB	partial weight bearing
q	every
qd	every day; daily
qh	every hour (or fill in hour [e.g., q4h])
qid	four times a day
qod	every other day
R	rectal
RA	room air
R*A*C*E	**R**escue individuals in danger; **A**larm—sound the alarm; **C**onfine the fire by closing all doors and windows; **E**xtinguish the fire with the nearest suitable fire extinguisher
RBC	red blood cell
RBS	random blood sugar
RD	registered dietitian
RDW	red cell distribution width
reg	regular
Retics	reticulocytes (hematology)
RIS	radiology information system
RL	Ringer's lactate
RLE	right lower extremity
RLL	right lower lobe
RLQ	right lower quadrant
R&M	routine and microscopic
RML	right middle lobe
RN	registered nurse
R/O	rule out
ROM	range of motion
Rout	routine
RPR	rapid plasmin reagin
RR	recovery room
	respiratory rate
RSV	respiratory syncytial virus
RT	respiratory therapist
Rt	routine
rt or ®	right
RUE	right upper extremity
RUL	right upper lobe
RUQ	right upper quadrant
Rx	take (e.g., treatment, medication)
s̄	without
s̊s̊	semis (one-half)
S&A	sugar and acetone (urinalysis)
SAD	save a day

Abbreviation	Meaning
SaO_2 or O_2 sats	oxygen saturation
SBFT	small bowel follow-through
SBU	small business unit
SC, sq, or sub-q	subcutaneous
SCD	sequential compression device
SDS	same-day surgery
SEP	somatosensory evoked potential
SHUC	student health unit coordinator
SICU	surgical intensive care unit
SIDS	sudden infant death syndrome
SL	sublingual
SNAT	suspected nonaccidental trauma
SNF	skilled nursing facility
SO_4	sulfate
SOB	shortness of breath
sol'n	solution
SOS	if needed (one dose only)
SSE	soap suds enema
SSU	short-stay unit
st	straight
stat	immediately
STM	soft tissue massage
subling, SL	sublingual (under the tongue)
supp	suppository
Surg	surgery
SVN	small volume nebulizer
syr	syrup
T_3, T_4, T_7	thyroid tests
T&A	tonsillectomy and adenoidectomy
tab	tablet
TAH	total abdominal hysterectomy
TB	tuberculosis
TBD	to be done
TBT	template bleeding time
T&C or T&X-match	type and crossmatch
TCDB	turn, cough, deep breathe
TCT or TT	thrombin clotting time or thrombin time
TDWB	touchdown weight bearing
Ted	antiembolism stockings
temp	temperature
TENS	transcutaneous electrical nerve stimulation
THR or THA	total hip replacement/total hip arthroplasty
TIA	transient ischemic attack
TIBC	total iron-binding capacity (chemistry)
TICU	trauma intensive care unit
tid	three times a day

Abbreviation	Meaning
Timed Specimen	to be drawn at specified time
tinct or tr	tincture
TJC	The Joint Commission
TKO	to keep open
TKR or TKA	total knee replacement/total knee arthroplasty
TPN	total parenteral nutrition
TPR	temperature, pulse, respiration
TRA	to run at
Trig or TG	triglycerides (chemistry)
T&S	type and screen
TSH	thyroid-stimulating hormone
T/stat	timed stat
TT	tilt table
TTOT	transtracheal oxygen therapy
TTWB	toe-touch weight bearing
TUR	transurethral resection
TWE	tap water enema
Tx	traction or treatment
U	unit
UA or U/A	urinalysis
UC	urine culture
UCR	usual, customary, and reasonable
UD	unit dose
UGI	upper gastrointestinal
ung	unguent (ointment)
US	ultrasound
USN	ultrasonic nebulizer
VAD	venous access device
VDRL	Venereal Disease Research Laboratories
VDT	video display terminal
VEP	visual evoked potential
vib & perc	vibration and percussion
VMA	vanillylmandelic acid
VNS	visiting nurse service
VS	vital sign
WA or W/A	while awake
WBAT	weight bearing as tolerated
WBC	white blood cell
WHO	World Health Organization
wk	week
WNL	within normal limits
WP	whirlpool
wt	weight
www	World Wide Web
X-match	crossmatch
Zn	zinc

Word Parts

Each word element present in Chapter 23 of *LaFleur Brooks' Health Unit Coordinating*, 6th edition, is noted in **bold text**, along with its meaning and the unit of Chapter 23 in which it is found. Additional word parts that you may encounter in your medical work are provided in normal text, and instead of the unit number, a sample medical term that incorporates the word part is provided.

Word Element	Meaning	Unit Number (or Sample Medical Term)
a	without	1
abdomin / o	abdomen	7
-ac	pertaining to	*cardiac*
acou / o	hearing	*acoumeter*
acr / o	extremities, height	*acromegaly*
aden / o	gland	11
adren / o	adrenal	11
adrenal / o	adrenal	11
-al	pertaining to	2
-algia	pain	3
amnion / o	amnion, amniotic fluid	*amnionitis*
an-	without	1
angi / o	blood vessel	6
aort / o	aorta	6
-apheresis	removal	*plasmapheresis*
appendic / o	appendix	7
-ar	pertaining to	3
arteri / o	artery	6
arthr / o	joint	3
-ary	pertaining to	*pulmonary*
-asthenia	weakness	*myasthenia*

Word Element	Meaning	Unit Number (or Sample Medical Term)
atel / o	imperfect, incomplete	*atelectasis*
ather / o	yellowish, fatty plaque	*atherosclerosis*
-atresia	absence of normal body opening, occlusion	*hysteratresia*
aut / o	self	*autopsy*
balan / o	glans penis	*balanitis*
bi-	two	*bilateral*
blephar / o	eyelid	5
brady-	slow	6
bronch / o	bronchus	8
cancer / o	cancer	2
carcin / o	cancer	2
cardi / o	heart	2
caud / o	tail or down	*caudal*
-cele	herniation, protrusion	4
-centesis	surgical puncture to aspirate fluid	4
cerebell / o	cerebellum	4
cerebr / o	cerebrum	4
cervic / o	cervix	10
cheil / o	lip	7
cholangi / o	bile duct	*cholangioma*
chol / e, chol / o	bile, gall	7
choledoch / o	common bile duct	*choledocholithiasis*
chondr / o	cartilage	3
clavic / o	clavicle	3
clavicul / o	clavicle	3
-coccus	berry-shaped (form of bacterium)	*Staphylococcus*
col / o	colon	7
colp / o	vagina	10
conjunctiv / o	conjunctiva	5
cost / o	rib	3
crani / o	cranium	3
crypt / o	hidden	*onychocryptosis*
cutane / o	skin	2
cyan / o	blue	6
cyst / o	bladder, sac	7, 9
-cyte	cell	*erythrocyte*
cyt / o	cell	1, 2
derm / o	skin	2
dermat / o	skin	2
diverticul / o	diverticulum	*diverticulosis, diverticulitis*
duoden / o	duodenum	7

Word Element	Meaning	Unit Number (or Sample Medical Term)
dys-	difficult, labored, painful, abnormal	8
ech / o	sound	*echocardiogram*
-ectasis	expansion	*atelectasis*
-ectomy	excision, surgical removal	1, 3
electr / o	electricity, electrical activity	1, 3
-emia	condition of the blood	6
encephal / o	brain	4
endo-	within	6
enter / o	intestine	7
epididym / o	epididymis	*epididymitis*
episi / o	vulva	*episiotomy*
epitheli / o	epithelium	2
erythr / o	red	6
esophag / o	esophagus	7
eti / o	cause (of disease)	etiology
femor / o	femur	3
fibr / o	fiber	*fibromyalgia*
gastr / o	stomach	7
-genic	producing, originating, causing	2
gloss / o	tongue	7
-gram	record, x-ray image	3
-graph	instrument used to record	3
-graphy	process of recording, x-ray imaging	3
gravid / o	pregnancy	*gravida*
gynec / o	woman	10
hem / o	blood	6
hemat / o	blood	6
hepat / o	liver	7
herni / o	protrusion of a body part	7
hist / o	tissue	2
humer / o	humerus	3
hyper-	above normal	6
hypo-	below normal	6
hyster / o	uterus	10
-ial	pertaining to	*endometrial*
-iasis	condition of	7
-iatrist	specialist, physician	*physiatrist*

Word Element	Meaning	Unit Number (or Sample Medical Term)
iatr / o	physician, treatment	*iatrogenic*
-ic	pertaining to	3
-ior	pertaining to	*posterior*
ile / o	ileum	7
inter-	between	*intervertebral*
intra-	within	1
irid / o	iris	5
isch / o	deficiency, blockage	*ischemia*
-itis	inflammation	3
kal / i	potassium	*hyperkalemia*
kerat / o	cornea	5
labyrinth / o	labyrinth	*labyrinthitis*
lact / o	milk	*lactorrhea*
lamin / o	lamina	3
lapar / o	abdomen	7
laryng / o	larynx	8
lei / o	smooth	*leiomyosarcoma*
leuk / o	white	6
lingu / o	tongue	7
lip / o	fat	2
lith / o	stone, calculus	7
-logist	one who specializes in the diagnosis and treatment of	2
-logy	study of	2
-lysis	loosening, dissolution, separating	*urinalysis*
-malacia	softening	*chondromalacia*
mamm / o	breast	10
mast / o	breast	10
-megaly	enlargement	6
melan / o	black	*melanoma*
men / o	menstruation	10
mening / o	meninges	4
menisc / o	meniscus	3
meta-	after, beyond, change	*metastasis*
-meter	instrument used to measure	*spirometer*
metr / o	uterus	10
-metry	measurement	*pelvimetry*
myc / o	fungus	*onychomycosis*
my / o	muscle	3
myel / o	spinal cord, bone marrow	4

Word Element	Meaning	Unit Number (or Sample Medical Term)
myring / o	tympanic membrane	5
nat / o	birth	*prenatal*
natr / o	sodium	*hyponatremia*
necr / o	death (cells, body)	*necrosis*
neo-	new	*neonatal*
nephr / o	kidney	9
neur / o	nerve	4
noct / i	night	*nocturia*
-odynia	pain	*cardiodynia*
-oid	resembling	2
olig / o	scanty, few	*oliguria*
-oma	tumor	2
onc / o	cancer	2
onych / o	nail	*onychomalacia*
oophor / o	ovary	10
ophthalm / o	eye	5
-opsy	to view	*biopsy*
orchi / o	testicle, testis	9
orchid / o	testicle, testis	9
organ / o	organ	*organic*
-osis	abnormal condition	3
oste / o	bone	3
ot / o	ear	5
-oxia	oxygen	*hypoxia*
-ous	pertaining to	2
pancreat / o	pancreas	7
parathyroid / o	parathyroid	11
part / o	give birth to, labor, childbirth	*parturition*
patell / o	patella	3
path / o	disease	2
-pathy	disease	*neuropathy*
peri-	surrounding (outer)	6
perine / o	perineum	10
-pexy	surgical fixation	6
-phagia	swallowing	*dysphagia*
phalang / o	phalange	3
pharyng / o	pharynx	8
phas / o	speech	4
phleb / o	vein	6
-phobia	fear of	*claustrophobia*
phot / o	light	*photophobia*
-plasty	surgical repair	3
-plegia	paralysis, stroke	4

Word Element	Meaning	Unit Number (or Sample Medical Term)
pleur / o	pleura	8
-pnea	respiration, breathing	8
pneum / o	air, lung	8
pneumon / o	lung	8
-poiesis	formation	*hematopoiesis*
poli / o	gray matter	4
prim / i	first	*primigravida*
proct / o	rectum	7
prostat / o	prostate	9
psych / o	mind	4
-ptosis	drooping, sagging, prolapse	*nephroptosis*
puerper / o	childbirth	*puerperal*
pulmon / o	lung	8
pyel / o	renal pelvis	9
pylor / o	pylorus, pyloric sphincter	*pyloroplasty*
quadr / i	four	*quadriplegia*
radic / o	nerve root	*radiculitis*
radicul / o		
rhiz / o		
ren / o	kidney	9
retin / o	retina	5
rhabd / o	rod-shaped, striated	*rhabdomyolysis*
rhin / o	nose	8
-rrhagia	rapid flow of blood	4
-rrhaphy	surgical repair	4
-rrhea	excessive discharge, flow	4
-rrhexis	rupture	*hysterorrhexis*
salping / o	fallopian or uterine tube	10
sarc / o	connective tissue, flesh	2
-sarcoma	malignant tumor	*rhabdomyosarcoma*
scapul / o	scapula	3
scler / o	sclera, hard	5
-sclerosis	hardening	6
-scope	instrument used for visual examination	3
-scopic	pertaining to visual examination	*arthroscopic*
-scopy	visual examination	3
sigmoid / o	sigmoid colon	7
-sis	state of	*diagnosis*
son / o	sound	*sonogram*

Word Element	Meaning	Unit Number (or Sample Medical Term)
somat / o	body	*psychosomatic*
-spasm	involuntary muscle contraction	*bronchospasm*
spin / o	spine	4
splen / o	spleen	6
staped / o	stapes	5
staphyl / o	grape-like clusters	*Staphylococcus*
-stasis	control, stop, standing	*metastasis*
-stenosis	narrowing	6
stern / o	sternum	3
stomat / o	mouth	7
-stomy	creation of an artificial opening	7
streptococcus	twisted chains	*Streptococcus*
sub-	under, below	1
supra-	above	*suprascapular*
tachy-	fast, rapid	6
thorac / o	chest	8
-thorax	chest	*pneumothorax*
thromb / o	clot	6
thyr / o	thyroid	11
thyroid / o	thyroid	11
tom / o	cut, section	*tomogram*
-tomy	surgical incision or to cut into	3
tonsill / o	tonsil	8
trache / o	trachea	8
trans-	through, across, beyond	1
trich / o	hair	2
-trophy	development, nourishment	3
ungu / o	nail	2
ur / o	urine, urinary tract	9
ureter / o	ureter	9
urethr / o	urethra	9
uria-	urine, urination	*albuminuria*
urin / o	urine	9
uter / o	uterus	10
vagin / o	vagina	10
vas / o	vessel, duct	9
ven / o	vein	6
vertebr / o	vertebra	3
viscer / o	internal organs	2

Medical/Diagnostic/ Surgical Terms

Terms in this appendix are divided into four sections: medical/general, surgical procedures, disease/conditions and diagnostic procedure terms, and surgical abbreviations.

Medical/General Terms

Term	Meaning
abdominal (ăb-dŏm'-ĭn-al)	pertaining to the abdomen
adenitis (ăd-ĕ-nī i'-tĭs)	inflammation of a gland
adenoids (ăd'-ĕn-oyds)	tissue in the nasopharynx
adenoma (ăd-ĕ-nō'-mah)	a tumor of glandular tissue
adenosis (ăd-ĕ-nō'-sĭs)	disease of a gland
adrenal (ah-drē'-nal)	adrenal gland
adrenalitis (ah-drē-năl-ī'-tĭs)	inflammation of the adrenal gland
aortic (ā-or'-tĭk)	pertaining to the aorta
aphasia (ah-fā'-zē-ah)	without speech
apnea (ăp'-nē-ah)	absence of breathing
arrhythmia (ah-rĭth'-mē-ah) (heart)	irregular heartbeat
atrophy (ăt'-rō-fē)	without development
bradycardia	condition of slow heart (rate)
bronchotracheal (brŏn'-kō-trā'-kē-al)	pertaining to the bronchi and trachea
carcinogenic (kar'-sĭn-ō-jĕn'-ik)	producing cancer
cardiac arrest (kar'-dē-ăk) (ah-rĕst')	sudden and often unexpected stoppage of the heartbeat
cardiologist (kar-dē-ŏl'-o-jĭst)	one who specializes in cardiology

Term	Meaning
cardiology (kar-dē-ŏl′-o-jē)	the study of the heart (and its functions and diseases)
cardiomegaly (kar′-dē-ō-mĕg′-ah-lē)	enlargement of the heart
cardiovascular (kar′-dē-ō-văs′-kū-lar)	pertaining to the heart and blood vessels
cerebrospinal (ser′-ē-brō-spī′-nal)	pertaining to the brain and spine
chondrogenic (kŏn-drō-jĕn′-ĭk)	producing cartilage
coronary (kŏr′-ō-nā-rē)	pertaining to the heart
cranial (krā′-nē-al)	pertaining to the cranium
cytoid (sī′-toyd)	resembling a cell
cytology (sī-tŏl′-o-jē)	study of cells
dermal (dĕr′-mal)	pertaining to the skin
dermatoid (dĕr′-măh-toyd)	resembling skin
dermatologist (dĕr-măh-tŏl′-o-jĭst)	one who specializes in dermatology
dermatology (dĕr-măh-tŏl′-o-jē)	study of skin (branch of medicine that deals with diagnosis and treatment of skin disease)
diarrhea (dī′-ah-rē′-ah)	frequent discharge of watery stool
duodenal (doo-ō-dē′-nal)	pertaining to the duodenum
dysentery (dĭs′-ĕn-tĕr-ē)	inflammation of the intestine
dyspnea (dĭsp-nē′-ah)	difficulty in breathing
dystrophy (dĭs′-trō-fē)	abnormal development
endocardial (ĕn-dō-kar′-dē-al)	pertaining to within the heart
endotracheal (ĕn-dō-trā′-kē-al)	pertaining to within the trachea
epithelial (ĕp-ĭ-thē′-lē-al)	pertaining to epithelium
erythrocyte (ē-rĭth′-rō-sīt)	red (blood) cell (RBC)
femoral (fĕm′-ō-ral)	pertaining to the femur (or thigh bone)
gland	a secretory organ that produces hormones or other substances
glossoplegia (glŏss-ō-plē′-ja)	paralysis of the tongue
gynecologist (gī-nĕ-kŏl′-o-jĭst)	specialist in gynecology
gynecology (gī-nĕ-kŏl′-o-jē)	study of women (the branch of medicine dealing with diseases and disorders of the female reproductive system)
hematuria (hēm-ah-tū′-rē-ah)	blood in the urine
hemiplegia (hĕm-ĭ-plē-ja)	paralysis of the right or left side of the body

Term	**Meaning**
hemorrhage (hĕm'-ō-rĭj)	the rapid flow of blood (from a blood vessel)
hepatoma (hep-ah-tō'-mah)	a tumor of the liver
hepatomegaly (hĕp'-ah-tō-mĕg'-ah-lē)	enlargement of the liver
hernia (her'-nē-ah)	an abnormal protrusion of a body part through the containing structure
histology (hĭs-tŏl-o-jē)	study of tissues
hormones	chemical messengers produced by the endocrine system
humeral (hū'-mĕr-al)	pertaining to the humerus
hypertension (hī-per-tĕn'-shŭn)	high blood pressure
hypotension (hī-pō-tĕn'-shu˘n)	low blood pressure
intervertebral (ĭn-tĕr-vĕr'-tĕ-bral)	pertaining to between the vertebrae
intracranial (ĭn-trah-krā'-nē-al)	pertaining to within the cranium
intravenous (ĭn-trah-vē'-nŭs)	within a vein
jaundice (jawn'-dĭs)	yellowness of the skin and eyes; a symptom of hepatitis
leukocyte (loo'-kō-sīt)	white (blood) cell (WBC)
menopause (mĕn'-ō-pawz)	the period during which the menstrual cycle slows down and eventually stops
menstrual (mĕn'-stroo-ăl)	pertaining to menstruation
menstruation (mĕn-stroo-ā'-shŭn)	discharge of blood and tissue from the uterus, normally occurring every 28 days
myelorrhagia (mī-ĕ-lō-rā'-ja)	rapid flow of blood into spinal cord
neurologist (nū-rŏl'-o-jĭst)	one who specializes in neurology
neurology (nū-rŏl'-o-jē)	study of nerves (the branch of medicine that deals with the diagnosis and treatment of disorders or diseases of the nervous system)
oncology (ŏn-kol'-o-jē)	study of cancer
ophthalmologist (ŏf'-thal-mŏl'-o-jĭst)	one who specializes in the diagnosis and treatment of the eye (physician)
ophthalmology (ŏf'-thăl-mŏl'-o-jē)	study of the eye (and its diseases and disorders)

Term	Meaning
optometrist (ŏp-tŏm'-ĕ-trĭst)	a professional person trained to examine the eyes and prescribe glasses
orthopedics (or-thō-pē'-dĭks)	branch of medicine dealing with the diagnosis and treatment of disease, abnormalities, or fractures of the musculoskeletal system
orthopedist (or-thō-pē'-dist)	a doctor who specializes in orthopedics
osteoma (ŏs-tē-ō'-mah)	a tumor (composed of) bone
otorrhea (ō-tō-rē'-ah)	discharge from the ear
ovum (ō'-vŭm) (sing.); ova (ō'-vă) (pl.)	female reproductive cell
pancreatic (păn-krē-ăt'-ĭk)	pertaining to the pancreas
paraplegia (păr-ăh-plē'-ja)	paralysis of the legs and sometimes the lower part of the body
pathogenic (păth-ō-jĕ n'-ĭk)	producing disease
pathologist (pă-thŏl'-o-jĭst)	one who specializes in the diagnosis and treatment of disease (body changes caused by disease)
pathology (pă-thŏl'-o-jē)	the study of disease
pharyngocele (fah-rĭng'-gō-sēl)	(an abnormal) protrusion in the pharynx
pharyngoplegia (fah-rĭng-gō-plē'-ja)	paralysis of the pharynx
phlebotomy (flĕ-bŏt'-o-mē)	incision into the vein (to withdraw blood)
proctorrhea (prŏk-tō-rē'-ah)	excessive discharge from the rectum
pulmonary (pŭl'-mŏ-nĕr-ē)	pertaining to the lungs
quadriplegia (kwăd-rĕ-plē'-ja)	paralysis that affects all four limbs
scrotum (scrō'-tŭm)	the skin-covered sac that contains the testes and their accessory organs
secretion (sē-krē'-shŭn)	a substance produced by a gland
splenomegaly (splē-nō-mĕg'-ah-lē)	enlargement of the spleen
sternal (stĕr'-nal)	pertaining to the sternum
sternoclavicular (stĕr'-nō-klah-vĭk'-ū-lar)	pertaining to the sternum and clavicle

Term	**Meaning**
sternocostal (stĕr-nō-kŏs′-tal)	pertaining to the sternum and ribs
sternoid (stĕr′-noyd)	resembling the sternum
stomatogastric (stō′-mah-tō-găs′-trĭk)	pertaining to the mouth and stomach
subcostal (sŭb-kŏs′-tal)	pertaining to below a rib or ribs
subcutaneous	pertaining to under the skin
sublingual (sŭb-lĭng′-gwal)	pertaining to under the tongue
subscapular (sŭb-skăp′-ū-lar)	pertaining to below the scapula
subungual	pertaining to under the nail
suprascapular (soo-prah-skăp′-ū-lar)	pertaining to above the scapula
tachycardia (tăk-ē-kar′-dē-ah)	condition of rapid heart (rate)
thoracic (thō-răs′-ĭk)	pertaining to the chest
thoracocentesis (thō′-rah-kō-sĕn-tē′-sĭs) or thoracentesis	surgical puncture to remove fluid from the chest
thrombosis (thrŏm-bō′-sĭs)	abnormal formation of a blood clot
tracheoesophageal (trā′-kē-ō-ē-sŏf-ah-jē′-al)	pertaining to the trachea and esophagus
transdermal (trăns-dĕr′-mal),	pertaining to (entering) through the skin or transcutaneous
trichoid (trĭk′-oyd)	resembling hair
ulcer (ŭl′-ser)	a sore of the skin or mucous membrane
ureterovaginal (ū-rē′-ter-ō-văj′-ĭ-nal)	pertaining to the ureter and vagina
urethral (ū-rē′-thral)	pertaining to the urethra
urinary (ū′-rĭ-nĕr-ē)	pertaining to urine
urinary catheterization (kăth′-ĕ-ter-ĭ-zā′-shŭn)	insertion of a sterile tube through the urethra into the bladder to remove urine
urination (ū-rĭ-nā′-shŭn) or micturition	passage of urine from the body
urologist (ū-rŏl′-o-jĭst)	one who specializes in urology
urology (ū-rŏl′-o-jē)	study of the urinary tract; treatment of diseases of the male and female urinary tract and of the male reproductive organs

Term	Meaning
uterine (ū'-ter-ĭn)	pertaining to the uterus
vaginal (văj'-ĭ-nal)	pertaining to the vagina
vaginoperineal (văj-ĭ-nō- pĕr-ĭ-nē'-al)	pertaining to the vagina and perineum
vertebrocostal (vĕr'-tĕ-brō-kŏs'-tal)	pertaining to the vertebrae and ribs
visceral (vĭs'-er-al)	pertaining to internal organs
void (voyd)	to pass urine or feces from the body (usually refers to urine)

Surgical Procedure Terms

Term	Meaning
abdominal herniorrhaphy (ăb-dŏm'-ĭn-al) (her-nē-ōr'-ah-fē)	suturing of a weak spot or opening in the abdominal wall to prevent protrusion of organs
adenoidectomy (ăd'-ĕ-noy-dĕk'-to-mē)	surgical removal of the adenoids
angioplasty	surgical repair of a blood vessel
angiorrhaphy (ăn-jĕ-ōr'-ah-fē)	suturing of a blood vessel
appendectomy (ăp-ĕn-dĕk'-to-mē)	excision of the appendix
arthroplasty (ar'-thrō-plăs-tē)	surgical repair of a joint
arthrotomy (ar-thrŏt'-o-mē)	surgical incision of a joint
biopsy	removal of tissue or cells for examination
blepharoplasty (blĕf'-ah-rō-plăs-tē)	surgical repair of the eyelid
blepharorrhaphy (blĕf'-ah-rōr'-ah-fē)	suturing of an eyelid
carotid endarterectomy	surgical procedure to remove blockage from the carotid arteries
cataract extraction (kăt'-ah-răkt) (ĕk-străk'-shŭn)	removal of the clouded lens of the eye
cecocolostomy	surgical procedure that creates an anastomosis between the cecum and the colon
cecoileostomy	surgical procedure that connects the ileum with the cecum
cecopexy	surgical procedure to suspend the cecum to correct its excessive mobility

Term	**Meaning**
cecostomy	creation of an artificial opening into the cecum
cervicectomy (sĕr-vĭ-sĕk′-to-mē)	excision of the cervix
cesarean section	delivery of a baby by an incision through the mother's abdomen and uterus
cheiloplasty (kī′-lō-plăs-tē)	surgical repair of the lip
cholecystectomy (kō-lē-sĭs-tĕk′-to-mē) Note: *e* is used as the combining vowel between the word roots *chol* and *cyst*	excision of the gallbladder
chondrectomy (kŏn-drĕk′-to-mē)	excision of a cartilage
circumcision (sur′-kŭm-sĭzh′-ŭn)	surgical removal of the foreskin of the penis
clavicotomy (klăv-ĭ-kŏt′-o-mē)	surgical incision into the clavicle
colectomy (kō-lĕk′-to-mē)	excision of the colon
colostomy (kō-lŏs′-to-mē)	creation of an artificial opening into the colon
colporrhaphy (kōl-por′-ah-fē)	suturing of the vagina
coronary artery bypass graft	veins from under the arm and from the leg used to bypass a blocked coronary artery
corneal (kor′-nē-al) transplant	transplantation of a donor cornea into the eye of the recipient
costectomy (kŏs-tĕk′-to-mē)	excision of a rib
cranioplasty (krā′-nē-ō-plăs-tē)	surgical repair to the cranium
craniotomy (krā-nē-ŏt′-o-mē)	surgical incision into the cranium
debridement of wound	surgical removal of foreign material and/or damaged or infected tissue from a wound or burn
dilatation and curettage (D&C) (dīl-ah-tā′-shŭn) (kū-rĕ-tăhzh′)	surgical procedure to dilate the cervix and scrape the inner walls of the uterus (endometrium) for diagnostic and therapeutic purposes
endometrial ablation (en-dō mē′ trē al ab-lā′ shun)	use of laser to destroy endometrium in abnormal uterine bleeding
enucleation (ē-nū-klē-ā′-shŭn)	removal of an organ; often used to indicate surgical removal of the eyeball

Term	**Meaning**
esophagoenterostomy (ē-sŏf'-ah-gō-ĕn-ter-ŏs'-to-mē)	creation of an artificial opening between the esophagus and the intestines
gastrectomy (găs-trĕk'-to-mē); pyloroplasty (pī-lōr'-ō-plăs-tē); and vagotomy (vā-gŏt'-o-mē)	a surgical procedure performed for treatment of ulcers; gastrectomy is the removal of the stomach; pyloroplasty is the plastic repair of the pyloric sphincter; vagotomy is the incision into the vagus nerve, performed to reduce the amount of gastric juices in the stomach
gastric bypass (Roux-en-Y gastric bypass)	bariatric surgery (to treat obesity) in which a small pouch is created at the top of the stomach and adds a bypass around a segment of the stomach and small intestine
gastrostomy (găs-trŏs'-to-mē)	creation of an artificial opening into the stomach (for feeding purposes)
glossorrhaphy (glŏ-sŏr'-ah-fē)	suturing of the tongue
hemorrhoidectomy (hĕm-ō-roi-dĕk'-to-mē)	excision of hemorrhoids
herniorrhaphy (her-nē-ōr'-ah-fē) (diaphragmatic, femoral, hiatal, or umbilical)	surgical repair of a hernia
hysterectomy (hĭs-tĕ-rĕk'-to-mē)	surgical removal of the uterus
hysterosalpingo-oophorectomy (hĭs'-ter-ō-săl-pĭng'-gō-ō-ŏf -ō-rĕk'-to-mē)	excision of the uterus, uterine tubes, and ovaries
ileostomy (īl-ē-ŏs'-to-mē)	creation of artificial opening into the ileum
iridectomy (īr-ĭ-dĕk'-to-mē)	excision of (a part of) the iris
iridosclerotomy (īr-ĭ-dō-sklĕ-rŏt'-o-mē)	incision into the iris and sclera
keratotomy (kĕr-ah-tot'-o-mē)	incision into the cornea (radial keratotomy is done to correct myopia [nearsightedness])
laminectomy (lăm-ĭ-nĕk'-to-mē)	surgical removal of lamina

Term	**Meaning**
laparotomy (lăp-ah-rŏt′-o-mē)	incision into the abdominal wall
laryngectomy (lar-ĭn-jĕk′-to-mē)	excision of the larynx
lobectomy (lō-bĕk′-to-mē)	excision of a lobe of an organ (lung, brain, liver, or thyroid gland)
lumpectomy	surgical excision of a discrete lump (usually a tumor)
mammoplasty (măm′-ō-plăs-tē)	surgical repair of the breast(s) to enlarge (augmentation) or reduce (reduction) in size or to reconstruct after surgical removal of a tumor
mastectomy (măs-tĕk′-to-mē)	surgical removal of all or part of the breast
partial (segmental)	involves the removal of the breast and a large portion of the normal breast tissue around the breast cancer
total (simple)	removal of the entire breast, including the nipple, the areola, and most of the overlying skin, and may also remove some of the lymph nodes under the arm
modified radical	removal of the entire breast (including the nipple, the areola and the overlying skin), some lymph nodes under the arm, and the lining over the chest muscles
radical	involves removal of the entire breast (including nipple, the areola, and the overlying skin), the lymph nodes under the arm and the chest muscles
meniscectomy (mĕn-ĭ-sĕk′-to-mē)	excision of the meniscus (of the knee joint)
myringoplasty (mĭ-rĭng′-gō-plăs-tē)	surgical repair of the tympanic membrane
myringotomy (mĭ-rĭng-gŏt′-o-mē)	incision of the tympanic membrane
nephrectomy (nĕ-frĕk′-to-mē)	excision of the kidney

Term	Meaning
nephrolithotomy (nĕf'-rō-lĭ-thŏt'-o-mē)	incision into the kidney (to remove a stone)
nephropexy (nĕf'-rō-pĕk-sē)	surgical fixation of a kidney
neuroplasty (nū'-rō-plăs-tē)	surgical repair of a nerve
neurorrhaphy (nū-rŏr'-ah-fē)	suturing of a nerve
oophorectomy (ō-ŏf-ō-rĕk'-to-mē)	excision of an ovary; a *bilateral oophorectomy* is the excision of both ovaries
ophthalmectomy (ŏf-thal-mĕk'-to-mē)	excision of the eye
orchiectomy (ōr-kē-ĕk'-to-mē)	excision of (one or both) testes
parathyroidectomy (pār'-ah-th-ī-roy-dĕk'-to-mē)	excision of the parathyroid gland
patellectomy (păt-ĕ-lĕk'-to-mē)	excision of the patella
perineoplasty (pĕr-ĭ-nē'-ō-plăs-tē)	surgical repair of the perineum
perineorrhaphy (pĕr'-ĭ-nē-ōr'-ah-fē)	suturing of the perineum
pleuropexy (ploo'-rō-pĕk'-sē)	surgical fixation of the pleura
pneumonectomy (nū-mŏ-nĕk'-to-mē)	excision of the lung (total or partial)
prostatectomy (prŏs-tah-tĕk'-to-mē)	surgical removal of the prostate gland
rhinoplasty (rhī-nō-plăs'-tē)	surgical repair of the nose
salpingo-oophorectomy (săl-pĭng'-gō-ō-ŏf-o-rĕk'-to-mē)	excision of a fallopian tube and an ovary
salpingopexy (săl-pĭng'-gō-pĕk-sē)	surgical fixation of a fallopian tube
scleroplasty (sklĕ'-rō-plăs-tē)	surgical repair of the sclera
sclerotomy (skĕ-rŏt'-o-mē)	incision into the sclera
skin graft	involves detaching healthy skin from one part of the body to repair areas of lost or damaged skin in another part of the body
splenectomy (splĕ-nĕk'-to-mē)	excision of the spleen
splenopexy (splĕ'-nō-pĕk-sē)	surgical fixation of the spleen
stapedectomy (stā-pē-dĕk'-to-mē)	excision of the stapes
thoracotomy (thō-rah-kŏt'-o-mē)	incision into the chest cavity
thyroidectomy (th-ī-roy-dĕk'-to-mē)	surgical removal of the thyroid gland
tonsillectomy (tŏn-sĭl-lĕk'-to-mē)	surgical removal of the tonsils
tracheostomy (trā-kē-ŏs'-to-mē)	artificial opening into the trachea (through the neck)

Term
transurethral resection of the prostate
gland (TURP)
(trăns-ū-rē'-thral) (rē-sĕk'-shŭn)
ureterolithotomy
(ū-rē'-ter-ō-lĭ-thŏt'-o-mē)
urethroplasty (ū-rē'-thrō-plăs'-tē)
urethrorrhaphy (ū-rē-thrōr'-ah-fē)
vasectomy (vah-sĕk'-to-mē)

vertebrectomy (vĕr-tĕ-brĕk'-to-mē)

Meaning
removal of a portion of the
prostate through the
urethra
incision into the ureter to
(remove) a stone
surgical repair of the urethra
suturing of a urethral tear
excision of a duct (vas
deferens or a portion of the
vas deferens; produces
sterility in the male)
excision of a vertebra

Disease/Condition Terms
Term
Addison's disease (ăd'-i-sŭnz)

adenoiditis (ăd'-ĕ-noy-dī-tĭs)
amenorrhea (ā-mĕn-ō-rē'-ah)
anemia (ah-nē'-mē-ah)

aneurysm (ăn'-ū-rĭzm)

appendicitis (ah-pĕn-dĭ-sī'-tĭs)
arteriosclerosis
(ar-tē'-rē-ō-sclĕ-rō'-sĭs)
arteriostenosis
(ar-tē'-rē-ō-stĕ-nō'-sĭs)
arthralgia (ar-thrăl'-ja)
arthritis (arthrī'-tĭs)
arthrosis (ar-thrŏ'-sĭs)
asthma (ăz'-mah)

bronchitis (brŏn-kī'-tĭs)
carcinoma (kăr-sĭ-nō'-mah)
cataract (kăt'-ah-răkt)

cerebellitis (ser-ĕ-bĕl-ī'-tĭs)

Meaning
disease caused by lack of
production of hormones by
the adrenal gland
inflammation of the adenoids
without menstrual discharge
condition of blood without
(deficiency in the number
of erythrocytes [RBC])
a dilation of a weak area of
the arterial wall
inflammation of the appendix
abnormal condition of
hardening of the arteries
abnormal condition of
narrowing of an artery
pain in a joint
inflammation of a joint
abnormal condition of a joint
chronic disease characterized
by periodic attacks of
dyspnea, wheezing, and
coughing
inflammation of the bronchi
cancerous tumor (malignant)
cloudiness of the lens
of the eye
inflammation of the
cerebellum

Term	**Meaning**
cerebral palsy (ser′-ē-bral) (paul′-zē)	partial paralysis and lack of muscle coordination from a defect, injury, or disease of the brain, which is present at birth or shortly thereafter
cerebrosis (ser-ĕ-brō′-sĭs)	abnormal condition of the brain
cerebrovascular accident (CVA) (ser′-ĕ-brō-văs′-kŭ-lăr)	impaired blood supply to parts of the brain; also called a stroke
cervicitis (ser-vĭ-sī′-tĭs)	inflammation of the cervix
cholecystitis (kō-lē-sĭs-tī′-tĭs)	inflammation of the gallbladder
cholelithiasis (kō-lē-lĭ-thī′-ah-sĭs) Note: *e* is used as the combining vowel between the word roots *chol* and *lith*	a condition of gallstones
chondritis (krŏn-drī′-tĭs)	inflammation of the cartilage
chronic obstructive pulmonary disease (COPD)	chronic obstruction of the airway that results from emphysema, asthma, or chronic bronchitis
congestive heart failure (CHF)	inability of the heart to pump sufficient amounts of blood to the body parts
conjunctivitis (kŏn-jŭnk-tī-vī′-tĭs)	inflammation of the conjunctiva (pinkeye)
coronary occlusion (kŏr′-ŏ-nā-rē) (ō-kloo′-zhŭn)	the closing off of a coronary artery, which usually results in damage to the heart muscle; commonly referred to as a heart attack
coronary thrombosis (kŏr′-ŏ-nā-rē) (thrŏm-bō′-sĭs)	the blocking of a coronary artery by a blood clot; commonly referred to as a heart attack
Crohn's (krōnz) disease	chronic inflammatory disease that can affect any part of the bowel, most often the lower small intestine
Cushing's disease (koosh′ĭngz)	a disorder caused by overproduction of certain hormones by the adrenal cortex
cystitis (sĭs-tī′-tĭs)	inflammation of the bladder
cystocele (sĭs′-tō-sēl)	herniation of the urinary bladder

Term	Meaning
dermatitis (dĕr-mah-tī′-tĭs)	inflammation of the skin
diabetes insipidus (dī-ah-bē′-tĭs) (ĭn-s—ĭp′-ĭ-dĭs)	disease caused by inadequate antidiuretic hormone production by the posterior lobe of the pituitary gland
diabetes mellitus (dī-ah-bē′-tĭs) (mĭl-ī′-tĭs)	disease that results in the inability of the body to store and use carbohydrates in the usual manner; it may be caused by inadequate production of insulin by the islets of Langerhans
diverticulitis (dī-ver-tĭk-ū-lī′-tĭs)	inflammation of the diverticula (small pouches in the intestinal wall)
duodenal ulcer (dū-ō-dē′-nal) (ŭl′-sĕr)	ulcer (sore open area) in the duodenum
dysmenorrhea (dĭs-mĕn-ō-rē′-ah)	painful menstrual discharge
edema (ĕ-dē′-mah)	an abnormal accumulation of fluid in the intercellular spaces of the body
embolism (ĕm′-bō-lĭzm)	a floating mass that blocks a vessel
emphysema (ĕm-fĭ-sē′-mah)	degenerative disease characterized by destructive changes in the walls of the alveoli, resulting in loss of elasticity to the lungs
encephalitis (ĕn-sĕf-ah-lī′-tĭs)	inflammation of the brain
encephalocele (ĕn-sĕf′-ah-lō-sēl)	herniation of brain (tissue through a gap in the skull)
endocarditis (ĕn-dō-kar-dī′-tĭs)	inflammation of the inner (lining) of the heart
epilepsy (ĕp′-ĭ-lĕp-sē)	convulsive disorder of the nervous system characterized by chronic or recurrent seizures
epithelioma (ĕp-ĭ-thē-lē-ō′-mah)	tumor (composed of) epithelial cells
gastric ulcer (găs′-trĭk) (ŭl′-ser)	ulcer pertaining to the stomach
gastritis (găs-trī′-tĭs)	inflammation of the stomach
glaucoma (glaw-kō′-mah)	an eye disease caused by increased pressure within the eye

Term	Meaning
hematology (hē-mah-tŏl′-o-jē)	study of the blood
hematoma (hē-mah-tō′-mah)	a tumor (-like mass) formed from blood (in the tissues)
hemophilia (hē-mō-fĭl′-ē-ah)	a congenital disorder characterized by excessive bleeding
hemorrhoid (hĕm′-ōrr-oyd)	enlarged vein in the rectal area
hepatitis (hĕp-ah-tī′-tĭs)	inflammation of the liver
hydrocele (hī′-drō-sēl)	scrotal swelling caused by the collection of fluid in the membrane covering the testes
hyperthyroidism (hī-per-thī′-roy-dĭzm)	excessive production of thyroxin and often an enlarged thyroid gland (goiter); also called Graves' disease or exophthalmic goiter
hypothyroidism (hī-pō-thī′-roy-dĭzm)	condition of underproduction of thyroxin by the thyroid gland
ileitis (ĭl-ē-ī′-tĭs)	inflammation of the ileum
infectious hepatitis (ĭn-fĕk′-shŭs) (hĕp-ah-tī′-tĭs)	inflammation of the liver (caused by a virus)
keratocele (kĕr′-ah-tō-sĕl)	herniation (of a layer) of the cornea
keratoconjunctivitis (kĕr′-ah-tō-kŏn-jŭnk-tĭ-vī′-tĭs)	inflammation of the cornea and conjunctiva
laryngitis (lar-ĭn-jī′-tĭs)	inflammation of the larynx
leukemia (loo-kē′-mē-ah)	a type of cancer characterized by rapid abnormal production of white blood cells
lipoma (lī-pō′-mah)	tumor (containing) fat
meningitis (mĕn-ĭn-jī′-tĭs)	inflammation of the meninges
meningomyelocele (mē-nĭng-gō-mī′-ē-lō-sĕl)	protrusion of the spinal cord and meninges (through the vertebral column)
meniscitis (mĕn-ĭ-sī′-tĭs)	inflammation of the meniscus (of the knee joint)
menometrorrhagia (mĕn-ō-mĕ-trō-rā′-ja)	rapid flow of blood from the uterus at menstruation (and in between menstrual periods)

Term	**Meaning**
metrorrhagia (mĕ-trō-rā′-ja)	rapid flow of blood from the uterus (bleeding at irregular intervals other than that associated with menstruation)
metrorrhea (mĕ-trō-rē′-ah)	(abnormal) uterine discharge
multiple sclerosis (MS) (mŭl′-tĭ-pl) (sklĕ-rō′-sĭs)	a degenerative disease of the nerves controlling muscles, characterized by hardening patches along the brain and spinal cord
muscular dystrophy (mŭs′-kū-lar) (dĭs′-trō-fē)	a number of muscle disorders characterized by a progressive, degenerative disease of the muscles
myocardial infarction (MI) (mī-ō-kar′-dē-al) (ĭn-fark′-shŭn)	damage to the heart muscle caused by insufficient blood supply to the area; a condition the lay person refers to as a heart attack
myoma (mī-ō′-mah)	a tumor (formed) of muscle (tissue)
nephritis (nĕ-frī′-tĭs)	inflammation of the kidney
nephrolithiasis (nĕf′-rō-lĭ-thī′-ah-sĭs)	a kidney stone
neuralgia (nū-răl′-ja)	pain in a nerve
neuritis (nū-rī′-tĭs)	inflammation of a nerve
neuroma (nū-rō′-mah)	a tumor made up of nerve (cells)
oophoritis (ō-ŏf-ō-rī′-tĭs)	inflammation of an ovary
otitis media (ō-tī′-tĭs) (mē′-dē-ah)	inflammation of the middle ear
pancreatitis (păn-krē-ah-tī′-tĭs)	inflammation of the pancreas
pericarditis (pĕr-ĭ-kar-dī′-tĭs)	inflammation of the outer (sac) of the heart (or pericardium)
pharyngitis (fah-rĕn-jī′-tĭs)	inflammation of the pharynx
pleuritis (ploo-rī′-tĭs); pleurisy (ploo′-rĕ-sē)	inflammation of the pleura
pneumonia (nū-mōn′-nē-ah)	inflammation or infection of the lung
pneumothorax (noo-mō-thor-ăks)	air in the pleural cavity causes the lung to collapse
poliomyelitis (pō′-lē-ō-mī-ĕ-lī′-tĭs)	inflammation of the gray matter of the spinal cord (virally caused disease, commonly known as *polio*)

Term	**Meaning**
pyelonephritis (pī'-ĕ-lō-nĕ-frī'-tĭs)	inflammation of the renal pelvis and kidney
renal calculus (rē'-nal) (kăl'-cū-lŭs)	a kidney stone
retinal detachment (rĕt'-ĭn-al) (dē-tăch'-mĕnt)	complete or partial separation of the retina from the choroid
rhinopharyngitis (rī'-nō-făr-ĭn-jī'-tĭs)	inflammation of the nose and throat
rhinorrhagia (rī-nō-rā'-ja)	bleeding from the nose, also called epistaxis
salpingitis (săl-pĭn-jī'-tĭs)	inflammation of a fallopian tube
salpingocele (săl-pĭng'-gō-sēl)	herniation of the fallopian tube
sarcoma (sar-kō'-mah)	tumor composed of connective tissue (highly malignant)
stomatitis (stŏ-mah-tī'-tĭs)	inflammation of the mouth
strabismus (străh-bĭz'-mŭs)	a weakness of the muscle of the eye (medical term for "crossed eyes")
subdural hematoma (sŭb-dū'-ral) (hēm-ah-tō'-mah)	blood tumor pertaining to below the dura mater (accumulation of blood in the subdural space)
thrombophlebitis (thrŏm'-bō-flĕ-bī'-tĭs)	inflammation of a vein (as the result of a clot)
tonsillitis (tŏn-sĭ-lī'-tĭs)	inflammation of the tonsils
tuberculosis (TB) (too-ber'kū-lō'-sĭs)	chronic infectious, inflammatory disease that commonly affects the lungs
ulcerative colitis (ul'-sĕ-ră-tĭv) (kō-lī'-tĭs)	inflammation of the colon with the formation of ulcers
upper respiratory infection (URI) (rĕ-spī'-rah-tō-rē)	infection of pharynx, larynx, or bronchi
uremia (ū-rē'-mē-ah)	urine in the blood (caused by inability of the kidneys to filter out waste products from the blood)
ureteralgia (ū-rē-ter-al'-ja)	pain in the ureter
ventricular fibrillation (VFib)	life-threatening uncoordinated contractions of the ventricles; immediate application of an electrical shock with a defibrillator is necessary treatment

Diagnostic Procedure Terms

Term	Meaning
abdominocentesis (ăb-doˇm′-ĭ-nō-sĕn-tē′-sĭs)	aspiration of fluid from the abdominal cavity
angiogram (ăn′-jē-ō-grăm)	an x-ray image of a blood vessel (using dye as a contrast medium)
aortogram (ā-ōr′-tō-grăm)	an x-ray image of the aorta (using dye as a contrast medium)
arteriogram (ar-tē′-rē-ō-grăm)	an x-ray image of an artery (using dye as a contrast medium)
arthrocentesis (ar-thrō-sĕn-tē′-sĭs)	surgical puncture to aspirate a joint
arthrogram (ar′-thrō-grăm)	x-ray image of a joint; (contrast medium, dye, or air is used)
arthroscope (ar′-thrō-scōpe)	instrument used to visualize a joint; (commonly the knee and shoulder)
arthroscopy (ar-thrŏs′-ko-pē)	visual examination of a joint (for diagnosing, identifying, and correcting problems)
barium enema (BE) (bă′-rē-ŭm) (ĕn′-ĕ-mah)	x-ray of the colon (fasting x-ray); barium is used as the contrast medium
blood glucose monitoring	method of monitoring the patient's glucose level by using a finger stick to obtain blood; performed by nursing staff
blood urea nitrogen (BUN)	laboratory test performed on a blood sample to determine kidney function
bronchogram (brŏn′-kō-grăm)	x-ray of the bronchi and lung (with the use of a contrast medium)
bronchoscope (brŏn′-kō-skōp)	instrument used to visually examine the bronchi
bronchoscopy (brŏn-kŏs′-ko-pē)	visual examination of the bronchi
cardiac catheterization (kar′-dē-ăk) (kăth′-ĕ-ter-ĭ-zā′-shŭn)	a diagnostic procedure to determine the presence of heart disease or heart defects

Term	Meaning
cervical Pap smear	a laboratory test used to detect cancerous cells in the cervix and uterus
cholangiogram (kō-lăn'-jē-ŏ-grăm)	x-ray image of the bile ducts (fasting x-ray)
colonoscope (kō-lŏn'-ō-skōp)	instrument used for visual examination of the colon
colonoscopy (kō-lŏn-ŏs'-ko-pē)	visual examination of the colon
colposcope (kŏl'-pō-skōp)	an instrument used for visual examination of the vagina and cervix
colposcopy (kŏl-pōs'-ko-pē)	visual examination of the vagina (and cervix)
creatinine (Cr)	laboratory test usually performed with the BUN to determine kidney function
CT scan (computed tomography)	use of radiologic imaging that produces cross-sectional pictures of the body
cystogram (sĭs'-tō-grăm)	x-ray image of the (urinary) bladder
cystoscopy (sĭs-tŏs'-ko-pē)	visual examination of the bladder
electrocardiogram (EKG) (ē-lĕk'-trō-kar'-dē-ō-grăm)	a record of the electrical activity of the heart
electrocardiograph (ē-lĕk'-trō-kar'-dē-ō-grăf)	instrument used to record electrical activity of the heart
electrocardiography (ē-lĕk'-trō-kar-dē-ŏg'-rah-fē)	the process of recording the electrical activity of the heart
electroencephalogram (EEG) (ē-lĕk'-trō-ĕn-sĕf'-ăh-lō-grăm)	record of the electrical activity of the brain
electromyogram (EMG) (ē-lĕk'-trō-mī'-ō-grăm)	record of electrical activity of a muscle
electromyography (ē-lĕk'-trō-mī'-ō-grăph)	instrument used to record the electrical activity of a muscle
electromyography (ē-lĕk'-trō-mī'-ŏg'-rah-fē)	process of recording the electrical activity of muscle
esophagogastroduodenoscopy (EGD) (ĕ-sŏf'-ah-gō-doo-odd-en-ŏs'-ko-pē)	visual examination of the esophagus, stomach, and and duodenum
esophagoscope (ĕ-sŏf'-ah-gō-skōp)	instrument used for the visual examination of the esophagus
esophagoscopy (ĕ-sŏf'-ah-gŏs'-ko-pē)	visual examination of the esophagus

Term	Meaning
fasting blood sugar (FBS)	laboratory test to determine the amount of glucose in the blood after patient has fasted for 8–10 hours
gastroscope (găs′-trō-skōp)	instrument used for the visual examination of the stomach
gastroscopy (găs-trŏs′-ko-pē)	visual examination of the stomach
hematocrit (hē′-măt-ō-krĭt)	laboratory test that measures the volume percentage of red blood cells in whole blood
hemoglobin (hē′-mō-glō′-bĭn)	the oxygen-carrying pigment of the red blood cells
hemoglobin A1C (Hb A1C)	laboratory test performed to more precisely determine the control of diabetes
hysterosalpingogram (hĭs′-ter-ō-săl-pĭng′-gō-grăm)	x-ray image of the uterus and fallopian tubes
intravenous pyelogram (IVP) (ĭn-trah-vē′-nŭs) (pī′-ĕ′-lō-grăm)	x-ray image of the kidney, especially the renal pelvis and ureters; contrast medium is used
kidneys, ureters, and bladder (KUB)	x-ray image of the kidneys, ureters, and bladder
laryngoscope (lăr-rĭng′-gō-skōp)	instrument for visual examination of the larynx
magnetic resonance imaging (MRI) nuclear magnetic resonance (NMR) imaging	a noninvasive procedure for taking pictures of the body by using powerful magnets and radio waves
mammogram (măm′-ō-grăm)	x-ray image of the breast
myelogram (mī′-ĕ-lō-grăm)	x-ray image of the spinal cord; (injected dye is used as the contrast medium)
ophthalmoscope (ŏf-thal′-mō-skōp)	instrument used for visual examination of the eye
otoscope (ō′-tō-skōp)	instrument used for visual examination of the ear
pneumoencephalogram (nū′-mō-ĕn-sĕf′-ăh-lō-grăm)	x-ray image (of the ventricles) in the brain using air (as the contrast medium)
proctoscope (prŏk′-tō-skōp)	instrument used for the visual examination of the rectum

Term	**Meaning**
proctoscopy (prŏk-tŏs′-ko-pē)	visual examination of the rectum
protein-bound iodine	laboratory test performed on a sample of blood to determine thyroid activity
sigmoidoscopy (sĭg-mol-dŏs′-ko-pē)	visual examination of the sigmoid colon
spinal puncture (tap) (lumbar puncture) (LP) (spī′-năl) (pŭngk′-chŭr)	the removal of cerebrospinal fluid (CSF) for diagnostic and therapeutic purposes
sternal puncture (stĕr′-nal) (pŭngk′-chŭr)	insertion of a hollow needle into the sternum to obtain a sample of bone marrow to be studied in the laboratory
T_3, T_4, and T_7 uptake	studies performed on a blood sample that use nuclear substances to determine the function of the thyroid gland
thoracentesis (thō-rah-sĕn-tē′-sĭs)	surgical puncture and drainage of fluid from the chest (cavity for diagnostic or therapeutic purposes)
thyroid scan	diagnostic study for thyroid gland function
upper gastrointestinal (UGI) (găs′-trō-ĭn-tĕs′-tĭ-nal)	x-ray of the esophagus and the stomach (fasting x-ray); barium is used as the contrast medium; UGI with small-bowel follow-through is an x-ray of the stomach and small intestines
urinalysis (UA) (ū-rĭ-năl′-ĭ-sĭs)	a laboratory test to analyze urine

Surgical Procedure Abbreviations

A&A	arthroscopy and arthrotomy
AKA	above the knee amputation
A&P repair	anterior and posterior colporrhaphy
A&P resection	abdominoperineal resection
AV fistula	arteriovenous fistula
AVR	aortic valve replacement
AV shunt	atrial/ventricular shunt
BKA	below the knee amputation
BSO	bilateral salpingo-oophorectomy
Bx	biopsy
CABG	coronary artery bypass graft

CR	closed reduction
D&C	dilation and curettage
DSA	diagnostic surgical arthroscopy
ECCE	extracapsular cataract extraction
EHL	electrohydraulic lithotripsy
ESWL	extracorporeal shock wave lithotripsy
EUA	examination under anesthesia
Exp Lap	exploratory laparotomy
FESS	fiberoptic endoscopic sinus surgery
FTSG	full-thickness skin graft
ICBG	iliac crest bone graft
LEEP	loop electrosurgical excision procedure
MMK	Marshall Marchetti Krantz
MMX	medial meniscectomy
MUA	manipulation under anesthesia
ORIF	open reduction, internal fixation
PEG	percutaneous endoscopic gastrostomy
PTCA	percutaneous transluminal coronary angioplasty
STSG	split-thickness skin graft
T&A	tonsillectomy and adenoidectomy
TAH	total abdominal hysterectomy
THR	total hip replacement
TKR	total knee replacement
TUIP	transurethral laser incision of the prostate
TURB	transurethral resection of the bladder
TURBN	transurethral resection of the bladder neck
TURP	transurethral resection of the prostate
TVH	total vaginal hysterectomy
TVR	tricuspid valve replacement
UPPP	uvulopalatopharyngoplasty
VATS	video-assisted thoracic surgery
	video-assisted thoracoscopic surgery

APPENDIX D

Commonly Ordered Medications

Generic Drug Name	Brand Name	Category
acetaminophen; butalbital; caffeine	Fioricet	Analgesic
acetaminophen; codeine	Tylenol; Codeine	Analgesic/Narcotic
acetaminophen; hydrocodone	Vicodin	Analgesic/Narcotic
acetaminophen; oxycodone	Endocet	Analgesic/Narcotic
acetaminophen; oxycodone	Percocet	Analgesic/Narcotic
acetaminophen; propoxyphene-N	Darvocet N	Analgesic/Narcotic
acetaminophen; tramadol	Ultracet	Analgesic
acyclovir	Zovirax	Antiviral
albuterol; ipratropium	Combivent	Bronchodilator
albuterol aerosol	Proventil	Bronchodilator
albuterol nebulizer solution	Proventil	Bronchodilator
alendronate	Fosamax	Bisphosphonate
allopurinol	Zyloprim	Antigout
alprazolam	Xanax	Sedative/Hypnotic
amikacin	Amikin	Antibiotic
amiodarone	Amiodarone HCL	Antiarrhythmic
amitriptyline	Elavil	Antidepressant
amlodipine	Norvasc	Calcium channel blocker
amlodipine; benazepril	Lotrel	Angiotensin
amoxicillin	Amoxil	Antibiotic
amoxicillin	Trimox	Antibiotic
amoxicillin; potassium clavulanate	Augmentin	Antibiotic

Generic Drug Name	Brand Name	Category
amoxicillin; potassium clavulanate	Augmentin ES-600	Antibiotic
amphetamine; dextroamphetamine extended-release	Adderall XR	Stimulant—central nervous system
aripiprazole	Abilify	Antipsychotic
aspirin; enteric-coated	Zorprin	Analgesic
atenolol	Tenormin	Beta blocker
atomoxetine	Strattera	Selective norepinephrine reuptake inhibitor
atorvastatin	Lipitor	Antihyperlipidemic
atropine sulfate	Atropine	Anticholinergic
azelastine	Astelin	H^1-receptor antagonist
azithromycin	Zithromax; Zithromax Z-Pak	Antibiotic
azithromycin	Zithromax Suspension	Antibiotic
baclofen	Azactam	Muscle relaxant
benazepril	Lotensin	Angiotensin
benzonatate	Tessalon Perles	Antitussive
benztropine	Cogentin	Antiparkinsonian
bisacodyl	Dulcolax	Laxative
bisoprolol; hydrochlorothiazide	Ziac	Beta blocker
brimonidine	Alphagan P	Adrenergic agonist
budesonide	Pulmicort	Inhaled antiinflammatory
budesonide nasal	Rhinocort Aqua	Corticosteroid
bupropion sustained-release	Wellbutrin SR	Antidepressant
buspirone hydrochloride	BuSpar	Antianxiety
candesartan	Atacand	Angiotensin
captopril	Capoten	Angiotensin
carbamazepine	Tegretol	Anticonvulsant
carbidopa	Sinemet	Antidyskinetic
carisoprodol	Soma	Muscle relaxant
carvedilol	Coreg	Beta blocker
cefaclor	Ceclor	Antibiotic
cefdinir	Omnicef	Antibiotic
cefprozil	Cefzil	Antibiotic

Generic Drug Name	Brand Name	Category
cefuroxime	Rocephin	Antibiotic
celecoxib	Celebrex	Analgesic/Antifungal
cephalexin	Keflex	Antibiotic
cetirizine	Zyrtec	Antihistamine
cetirizine; pseudoephedrine	Zyrtec-D	Antiallergy
cetirizine syrup	Zyrtec Syrup	Antihistamine
chlorhexidine gluconate	Peridex	Antiinfective
chlorpheniramine maleate	Chlor-Trimeton; Actifed	Antihistamine
chlorpromazine	Thorazine	Antiemetic/ Antipsychotic
ciprofloxacin	Cipro	Antiinfective
ciprofloxacin hydrochloride	Cipro	Antiinfective
citalopram	Celexa	Antidepressant
clobetasol	Temovate	Corticosteroid
clonazepam	Klonopin	Anticonvulsant
clonidine	Catapres	Antihypertensive
clopidogrel	Plavix	Platelet inhibitor
clotrimazole; betamethasone	Lotrisone	Antifungal
codeine; promethazine	Generic	Antiemetic/Antivertigo
colchicine		Antigout
cyclobenzaprine	Flexeril	Muscle relaxant
desloratadine	Clarinex	Antihistamine
desogestrel; ethinyl estradiol	Apri	Contraceptive
dextroamphetamine	Adderall XR	Stimulant
diazepam	Valium	Antianxiety
diclofenac sodium	Voltaren	Analgesic
dicyclomine hydrochloride	Bentyl	Anticholinergic
digoxin	Digitek	Antiarrhythmic
digoxin	Lanoxin	Antiarrhythmic
diltiazem CD	Cardizem	Antiarrhythmic
diltiazem extended release	Cartia XT	Antiarrhythmic
diphenoxylate hydrochloride	Lomotil	Antidiarrheal
divalproex sodium	Depakote	Anticonvulsant
docusate sodium	Colace	Laxative
donepezil	Aricept	Cholinesterase inhibitor
doxazosin	Cardura	Antiadrenergic
doxepin hydrochloride	Sinequan	Antidepressant
doxycycline	Vibramycin	Antibiotic

Generic Drug Name	Brand Name	Category
drospirenone; ethinyl estradiol	Yasmin 28	Contraceptive
duloxetine	Cymbalta	Antianxiety
enalapril	Vasotec	Angiotensin
enoxaparin	Lovenox	Anticoagulant
escitalopram	Lexapro	Antidepressant
esomeprazole	Nexium	Gastrointestinal
estradiol oral	Estrace	Hormone
estrogens conjugated	Premarin Tabs	Hormone
estrogens conjugated; medroxyprogesterone	Prempro	Hormone
eszopiclone	Lunesta	Hypnotic
ethinyl estradiol; levonorgestrel	Aviane	Hormone
ethinyl estradiol; levonorgestrel	Trivora-28	Contraceptive
etodolac	Lodine	Antiinflammatory
etonogestrel	NuvaRing	Contraceptive
ezetimibe	Zetia	Antihyperlipidemic
ethinyl estradiol; norelgestromin	Ortho Evra	Contraceptive
ethinyl estradiol; norgestimate	Ortho Tri-Cyclen	Contraceptive
famotidine	Pepcid	Gastrointestinal
felodipine	Plendil	Calcium channel blocker
fenofibrate	Tricor	Antihypertensive
fentanyl transdermal	Duragesic	Analgesic/Narcotic
ferrous sulfate	Hematinic	Iron supplement
fexofenadine	Allegra	Antihistamine
fexofenadine; pseudoephedrine	Allegra-D	Antihistamine
finasteride	Proscar	Hormone
fluconazole	Diflucan	Antifungal
fluoxetine	Prozac	Antidepressant
fluticasone	Flonase	Corticosteroid
fluticasone; salmeterol	Advair Diskus	Bronchodilator
fluticasone inhalation	Flovent	Corticosteroid
fluvastatin sodium	Lescol XL	Antihyperlipidemic
folic acid	Generic	Hematic
fosinopril	Monopril	Angiotensin
furosemide oral	Lasix	Diuretic
gabapentin	Neurontin	Anticonvulsant
gemfibrozil	Lopid	Antihyperlipidemic
glimepiride	Amaryl	Antidiabetic

Generic Drug Name	Brand Name	Category
glipizide	Glucotrol	Antidiabetic
glipizide extended release	Glucotrol XL	Antidiabetic
glyburide	Glycron	Antidiabetic
glyburide; metformin	Glucovance	Antidiabetic
heparin	Hepalean	Anticoagulant
human insulin isophane (recombinant)	Humulin N	Antidiabetic
human insulin regular/ isophane (recombinant)	Humulin 70/30	Antidiabetic
hydrochlorothiazide	HydroDIURIL	Diuretic
hydrocodone	Hycotuss expectorant	Cough suppressant
hydrocodone	Vicoprofin	Analgesic
hydrocortisone		Corticosteroid
hydroxychloroquine sulfate		Antiprotozoal
hydroxyzine	Atarax	Antiemetic/Antivertigo
hydroxyzine	Vistaril	Antihistamine
hyoscyamine	Anaspaz	Anticholinergic agent
ibuprofen	Advil	Analgesic
indomethacin	Indocin	Antiinflammatory
insulin aspart	Novolog	Antidiabetic
insulin glargine	Lantus	Antidiabetic
insulin lispro	Humalog	Antidiabetic
irbesartan	Avalide	Angiotensin
isosorbide mononitrate	Monoket	Nitrate/Vasodilator
isotretinoin	Accutane	Antiacne
ketoconazole	Nizoral	Antifungal
labetalol hydrochloride	Normodyne	Antiadrenergic
lamivudine	Epivir	Antiviral
lamotrigine	Lamictal	Anticonvulsant; Mood stabilizer (bipolar disorder)
lansoprazole	Prevacid	Gastrointestinal
latanoprost	Xalatan	Ophthalmic
levalbuterol hydrochloride	Xopenex	Bronchodilator
levofloxacin	Levaquin	Antiinfective
levothyroxine	Levothroid	Hormone
levothyroxine	Levoxyl	Hormone
levothyroxine	Synthroid	Hormone
lidocaine	Lidoderm	Local anesthetic
lisinopril	Zestril	Angiotensin
lisinopril; hydrochlorothiazide	Prinzide	Antihypertensive
lithium	Eskalith	Antipsychotic

Generic Drug Name	Brand Name	Category
loperamide	Imodium	Antidiarrheal
lorazepam	Ativan	Antianxiety
losartan	Cozaar	Angiotensin
losartan; hydrochlorothiazide	Hyzaar	Antihypertensive
lovastatin	Altocor	Antilipidemic
magnesium citrate	Citrate of Magnesia	Antidiarrheal
meclizine hydrochloride	Antivert	Antiemetic/Antivertigo
medroxyprogesterone tablets	Depo-Provera	Antineoplastic
meloxicam	Mobic	Antiinflammatory
memantine hydrochloride	Namenda	NMDA-receptor antagonist
meperidine hydrochloride	Demerol	Narcotic
metaxalone	Skelaxin	Muscle relaxant
metformin	Glucophage	Antidiabetic
metformin extended release	Glucophage XR	Antidiabetic
methadone	Methadose	Narcotic
methocarbamol	Robaxin	Muscle relaxant
methotrexate	Rheumatrex	Antineoplastic
methylphenidate	Ritalin	Stimulant—central nervous system
methylprednisolone tablets	Depo-Medrol	Corticosteroid
metoclopramide	Reglan	Antiemetic/Antivertigo
metoprolol succinate	Toprol XL	Beta blocker
metoprolol tartrate	Lopressor	Beta blocker
metronidazole tablets	Flagyl	Antiinfective
minocycline	Minocin	Antibiotic
mirtazapine	Remeron	Antidepressant
mometasone nasal	Nasonex	Corticosteroid
montelukast	Singulair	Antiasthmatic
morphine sulfate	Roxanol	Narcotic
moxifloxacin	Avalox	Antibacterial
moxifloxacin (ophthalmic)	Vigamox	Antibiotic
mupirocin	Bactroban	Antiinfective
nabumetone	Relafen	Analgesic
naproxen	Naprosyn	Analgesic/ Antiinflammatory
niacin	Niaspan	Antihyperlipidemic
nifedipine extended release	Procardia	Calcium channel blocker
nitrofurantoin	Macrobid	Antibiotic
nitroglycerin	Nitrek/Nitroquick	Vasodilator

Generic Drug Name	Brand Name	Category
norethindrone	Estrostep Fe	Estrogen/Progestin/Iron
nortriptyline	Aventyl HCl	Zanaflex
nystatin	Mycostatin	Antifungal
olanzapine	Zyprexa	Antipsychotic
olmesartan	Benicar	Angiotensin
olopatadine	Patanol	Antihistamine
omeprazole	Prilosec	Gastrointestinal
oseltamivir phosphate	Tamiflu	Antiviral
oxcarbazepine	Trileptal	Anticonvulsant
oxybutynin chloride extended release	Ditropan XL	Anticholinergic
oxycodone	OxyContin	Analgesic/Narcotic
pantoprazole	Protonix	Gastrointestinal
paroxetine	Paxil	Antidepressant
paroxetine hydrochloride controlled release	Paxil CR	Antidepressant
penicillin VK	Generic	Antibiotic
phenazopyridine hydrochloride	Urogesic	Urinary antiseptic
phenobarbital	Luminal	Anticonvulsant
phentermine	Adipex-P	Appetite suppressant
phenytoin sodium extended release	Dilantin	Anticonvulsant
phosphates	Fleets (enema/ Phospho-Soda)	Laxative
pimecrolimus	Elidel	Immuno- suppressive
pioglitazone	Actos	Antidiabetic
piroxicam	Feldene	Antiinflammatory
polyethylene glycol 3350	Miralax	Laxative
polyethylene glycol electrolyte sol	GoLYTELY	Laxative
potassium chloride	K-Dur; Klor-Con	Potassium replacement
pravastatin	Pravachol	Antihyperlipidemic
prednisolone	Cotolone	Corticosteroid
prednisone oral	Deltasone	Corticosteroid
progesterone	Prometrium	Hormone
promethazine tablets	Phenergan	Antiemetic/Antivertigo
propranolol hydrochloride	Inderal	Beta blocker
propranolol long acting	Inderal LA	Beta blocker
quetiapine	Seroquel	Antipsychotic
quinapril	Accupril	Angiotensin
rabeprazole	Aciphex	Gastrointestinal
raloxifene	Evista	Hormone

Generic Drug Name	Brand Name	Category
ramipril	Altace	Angiotensin
ranitidine hydrochloride	Zantac	Antihistamine
risedronate	Actonel	Bisphosphonate
risperidone	Risperdal	Antipsychotic
rofecoxib	Vioxx (withdrawn from the market in September 2004)	Analgesic/ Antiinflammatory
rosiglitazone	Avandia	Antidiabetic
rosuvastatin	Crestor	Antihyperlipidemic
senna	Senokot	Laxative
sertraline	Zoloft	Antidepressant
sildenafil	Viagra	Impotence agent
simvastatin	Zocor	Antihyperlipidemic
simvastatin	Vytorin	Antihyperlipidemic
spironolactone	Aldactone	Diuretic
sumatriptan oral	Imitrex Oral	Serotonin receptor agonist
tadalafil	Cialis	Impotence agent
tamoxifen citrate	Nolvadex	Antineoplastic
tamsulosin	Flomax	Alpha blocker
telithromycin	Ketek	Antibiotic
temazepam	Restoril	Sedative/Hypnotic
terazosin	Hytrin	Antiadrenergic
tervinafine hydrochloride	Lamisil	Antifungal
tetracycline	Brodspec	Antibiotic
thyroid	Armour Thyroid	Hormone
tiotropium bromide	Spiriva Handihaler	Anticholinergic
tizanidine hydrochloride	Zanaflex	Adrenergic agonist
tobramycin	Tobradex	Antibiotic
tolterodine long acting	Detrol LA	Anticholinergic
topiramate	Topamax	Anticonvulsant
tramadol	Ultram	Analgesic
trazodone hydrochloride	Desyrel	Antidepressant
triamcinolone acetonide nasal	Nasacort AQ	Corticosteroid
triamcinolone acetonide topical	Aristocort	Corticosteroid
triamterene; hydrochlorothiazide	Dyazide	Diuretic
trimethoprim/sulfa	Bactrim	Antibiotic
valacyclovir	Valtrex	Antiviral
valdecoxib	Bextra	Antiinflammatory
valsartan	Diovan	Angiotensin
valsartan; hydrochlorothiazide	Diovan HCT	Antihypertensive

Generic Drug Name	Brand Name	Category
vardenafil	Levitra	Impotence agent
venlafaxine extended release	Effexor XR	Antidepressant
ventolin inhalation	Albuterol	Bronchodilator
verapamil sustained release	Calan	Antiarrhythmic
warfarin	Coumadin	Anticoagulant
zafirlukast	Accolate	Antiasthmatic
zolpidem	Ambien	Sedative/Hypnotic

A Comprehensive List of Laboratory Studies and Blood Components

*The divisions indicated on this chart would be those found in a large hospital. Many hospitals combine bacteriology and virology into the Microbiology department. Space has been left at the end of each alphabetic section so that you can insert new tests as they are developed.

Procedure	Abbreviation	Laboratory Division	Specimen
ABO grouping (complete blood type)		Blood bank	Blood
Acetoacetic acid		Urinalysis	Urine
Acetone		Chemistry	Blood or urine
*Acid-fast culture	Culture for AFB (acid-fast bacilli)	Bacteriology	Sputum and tubercular lesions
*Acid-fast stain		Bacteriology	Sputum and tubercular lesions
Acid phosphatase	Acid Phos	Chemistry	Blood
Activated clotting time	ACT	Hematology/ POCT	Blood
Activated partial thromboplastin time	APTT	Hematology	Blood
Addis count		Urinalysis	Urine

POCT, Point-of-care testing. Some laboratory testing on blood, urine, and stool may be performed on the nursing unit.

Procedure	Abbreviation	Laboratory Division	Specimen
Adrenaline and noradrenaline (see Epinephrine and norepinephrine)			
Adrenocorticotropic hormone	ACTH	Chemistry	Blood
Alanine aminotransferase	ALT	Chemistry	Blood
Albumin	Alb	Chemistry	Blood or urine
Albumin/globulin ratio	A/G ratio	Chemistry	Blood
Alcohol (ethanol)		Chemistry	Blood
Aldolase		Chemistry	Blood
Aldosterone		Chemistry	Blood or urine
Alkaline phosphatase	ALP	Chemistry	Blood
Alkaline phosphatase isoenzymes		Chemistry	Blood
α_1-Antitrypsin		Chemistry	Blood
α_1-Fetoprotein		Chemistry	Blood
$17\alpha_1$-Hydroxypro-gesterone		Chemistry	Urine
Amino acids, fractionated		Chemistry	Urine
Ammonia	NH_3	Chemistry	Blood
Amniotic fluid		Chemistry	Amniotic fluid
Amoeba		Parasitology	Stool, cerebro-spinal fluid
Amphotericin level		Chemistry	Blood
Amylase		Chemistry	Blood or urine
Androstenedione		Chemistry	Urine
Angiotensin-converting enzyme	ACE	Chemistry	Blood
Ankylosing spondylitis (see HLA B27 typing)		Serology	Blood
Antideoxyribonuclease	DNA	Serology	Blood
Antidiuretic hormone	ADH	Chemistry	Blood
Antigen blood group (factor VIII)		Serology	Blood
Antimicrobial serum assay		Bacteriology	Blood
Antimony		Chemistry	Urine
Antinuclear antibody	ANA	Serology	Blood
Antistreptolysin O	ASO titer	Serology	Blood
Antithyroglobulin antibody		Serology	Blood

Procedure	Abbreviation	Laboratory Division	Specimen
Arsenic, quantitative		Chemistry	Urine
Ascorbic acid		Chemistry	Blood
Aspartate aminotransferase	AST	Chemistry	Blood
Barbiturates		Toxicology	Blood or urine
Basic metabolic panel	BMP	Chemistry	Blood
Bence Jones proteins	BJP	Chemistry	Urine
β-Hemolytic strep culture		Bacteriology	Nose or throat culture
$β_2$-Microglobulin		Chemistry	Blood
Bile		Urinalysis/ Chemistry	Urine or stool
Bilirubin (total and direct)	bili	Chemistry	Blood
Biopsy	bx	Pathology	All specimens
Bleeding time		Hematology	Blood
Blood culture	BC	Bacteriology	Blood
Blood sugar (BS) (glucose random)	RBS	Chemistry	Blood
Blood survey of coagulation defects		Hematology	Blood
Blood type (ABO and Rh)		Blood bank	Blood
Blood type and crossmatch	T&C, T&X-match	Blood bank	Blood
Blood urea nitrogen	BUN	Chemistry	Blood
Blood volume (Cr 51)		Chemistry	Blood
Blood volume (Risa)		Chemistry	Blood
Brain natriuretic peptide	BNP	Chemistry	Blood
Bromide		Chemistry	Blood
Bromsulphalein	BSP	Chemistry	Blood
Bronchial smear— Gram stain		Bacteriology	Bronchial smear
Brucella abortus		Serology	Blood
Buccal smear—sex chromosomes		Cytology	Buccal smear
Calcitonin		Chemistry	Blood
Calcium	Ca or Ca^+	Chemistry	Blood or urine
Calcium ionized		Chemistry	Blood
Capillary fragility		Hematology	Blood
Carbon dioxide	CO_2	Chemistry	Blood
Carbon monoxide	CO	Chemistry	Blood
Carboxyhemoglobin		Chemistry	Blood

Procedure	Abbreviation	Laboratory Division	Specimen
Carcinoembryonic antigen	CEA	Serology	Blood
Cardiac enzymes	CPK,CK-MB, AST, LDH, BNP, troponin	Chemistry	Blood
Carotene		Chemistry	Blood
Catecholamines (blood)		Chemistry	Blood
Catecholamines (urine)		Chemistry	Urine
Cell indices	RBC indices	Hematology	Blood
Cerebrospinal fluid (CSF) tests	CSF	Tests may be ordered from all divisions	Cerebrospinal fluid
Ceruloplasmin (see Ferroxidase)			
Cervical and vaginal smear	Pap test	Cytology	Cells from cervix and vagina
Chlamydia culture		Bacteriology	Swabs from specified areas
Chlamydia serology		Serology	Blood
Choral hydrate		Chemistry	Blood
Chloramphenicol level		Chemistry	Blood
Chloride	Cl	Chemistry	Blood, CSF, sweat, and urine
Cholesterol	Chol	Chemistry	Blood
Cholinesterase		Chemistry	Blood
Chorionic gonadotropin (serum)	hCG	Chemistry	Blood serum
Chorionic gonadotropin (urine)	hCG	Urinalysis	Urine
Chorionic gonadotropin (24-hour urine)	hCG	Chemistry	Urine 24-hour
Chromium 51 (blood volume)		Hematology	Blood

Procedure	Abbreviation	Laboratory Division	Specimen
Chromosome study (buccal smear)		Cytology	Buccal smear
Chromosome study		Chemistry	Blood—tissue
Citric acid		Chemistry	Urine
Clot retraction		Hematology	Blood
Clotting time (coagulation time)	Coag time or Lee-White	Hematology	Blood
CMV (cytomegalovirus) culture	CMV culture	Bacteriology	Blood or urine
CMV (cytomegalovirus) inclusions	CMV inclusions	Bacteriology	Blood or urine
CMV (cytomegalovirus) serology	CMV serology	Serology	Blood
Coagulation profile (platelets, APTT, prothrombin time, and bleeding time)		Hematology	Blood
Coagulation time, clotting time, thrombin clotting time, thrombin time	Coag time	Hematology	Blood
Cocci culture (fungus)	Coag time, TCT, TT	Mycology	Sputum
Coccidioides, complement fixation		Serology	Blood
Coccidioides, precipitin		Serology	Blood
Coccidioidomycosis— CSF titer		Serology	Cerebrospinal fluid
Cold agglutinins		Serology	Blood
Colloidal gold curve		Serology	Cerebrospinal fluid
Colony count	CC	Bacteriology	Body fluids
Complement	C_3	Chemistry	Blood
Complete blood count	CBC	Hematology	Blood
Complete urinalysis	UA	Urinalysis	Urine
Comprehensive metabolic panel	CMP	Chemistry	Blood
Coombs' test—direct/ indirect		Blood bank	Blood
Copper	CU	Chemistry	Blood
Coproporphyrins		Chemistry	Urine
Cord blood (grouping, Rh, and direct Coombs')		Blood bank	Blood
Corticosterone		Chemistry	Blood or urine

Procedure	Abbreviation	Laboratory Division	Specimen
Cortisol (compound F)		Chemistry	Blood or urine
Cortisol (compound S)		Chemistry	Blood or urine
C-reactive protein	CRP	Serology	Blood
Creatine		Chemistry	Blood
Creatine phosphokinase	CPK or CK	Chemistry	Blood
Creatinine		Chemistry	Blood and urine
Creatinine clearance	CC, creat cl, or cr cl	Chemistry	Blood and urine
Creatinine urine		Chemistry	Urine
Cryptococcus stain (India ink)		Microbiology	Cerebrospinal fluid
Culture and sensitivity	C&S	Bacteriology	Any body fluid
Cyanocobalamin (see Schilling test)			
Cystine		Chemistry	Urine
Cytology smears		Cytology	Any body cells
Cytotoxic antibodies		Blood bank	Blood
Dehydroepiandro-sterone	DHEA	Chemistry	Blood or urine
Deoxycorticosterone		Chemistry	Blood or urine
11-Deoxycortisols (compound S)		Chemistry	Blood or urine
Diacetic acid (see Acetoacetic acid)			
Differential cell count	Diff	Hematology	Blood
Digitoxin level		Chemistry	Blood
Digoxin level		Chemistry	Blood
Dihydrotestosterone	DHT	Chemistry	Blood
Dilantin level		Chemistry	Blood
Direct Coombs' (direct antiglobulin) test	DAT	Blood bank	Blood
Drug screen		Chemistry	Blood or urine
d-Xylose		Chemistry	Blood or urine
Electrolytes	Lytes-E'lytes	Chemistry/ POCT	Blood
Electrophoresis, Hb		Chemistry	Blood
Electrophoresis, Immuno		Chemistry	Blood
Electrophoresis, Lipids		Chemistry	Blood
Electrophoresis, Lipoprotein		Chemistry	Blood
Electrophoresis, protein	Protein ELP	Chemistry	Blood
Enterovirus		Virology	Stool

Procedure	Abbreviation	Laboratory Division	Specimen
Eosinophils		Hematology	Blood
Epinephrine and norepinephrine (catecholamines)		Chemistry	Urine
Epstein-Barr virus	EBV	Serology	Chemistry
Erythrocyte sedimentation rate	ESR	Hematology	Blood
Esophageal cytology		Cytology	Cells from esophagus
17β-Estradiol (E_2)		Chemistry	Urine
Estrogen receptor assay		Chemistry	Urine
Estrogens, E_1, E_2 (estrone, 17β-estradiol)		Chemistry	Urine
Ethyl alcohol, blood		Chemistry	Blood
Euglobulin clot lysis		Hematology	Blood
Factor assay (specify factor)		Hematology	Blood
Factor identifying test		Hematology	Blood
Fasting blood sugar (glucose, fasting)	FBS	Chemistry	Blood
Febrile agglutinins		Serology	Blood
Fecal fat, quantitative		Chemistry	Stool
Ferroxidase		Chemistry	Blood
Fibrin split product screen	FSP	Hematology	Blood
Fibrindex		Hematology	Blood
Fibrinogen level		Hematology	Blood
Fibrinolysin		Hematology	Blood
Fluorescent treponemal antibody	FTA	Serology	Blood
Folate (folic acid)		Chemistry	Blood
Follicle-stimulating hormone	FSH	Chemistry	Urine 24-hour
Fractionated alkaline phosphatase		Chemistry	Blood
Free fatty acids	FFA	Chemistry	Blood
Free thyroxine index	T_7	Chemistry	Blood
Fresh frozen plasma	FFP	Blood bank	Blood
Frozen cells		Blood bank	Blood
Frozen section	FS	Pathology	Any body tissue
Fungus culture		Bacteriology	Body specimen
Fungus serology		Serology	Blood

Procedure	Abbreviation	Laboratory Division	Specimen
Fungus smear		Mycology	Body specimen
Galactose, qualitative		Urinalysis	Urine
Gallium		Chemistry	Urine
Gastric analysis		Chemistry or GI lab	Gastric fluid
Gastric cytology		Cytology	Gastric fluid
Gastric washings (TB/ AFB)		Bacteriology	Gastric fluid
Gastrin		Chemistry	Blood
Gentamicin level		Toxicology	Blood
γ-Globulin (serum)		Chemistry	Blood
Globulin (total protein & albumin)		Chemistry	Blood
Glucose		Chemistry/ Urinalysis/ POCT	Blood or urine
Glucose (CSF)		Chemistry	Cerebrospinal fluid
Glucose, fasting	FBS	Chemistry	Blood
Glucose, 2-hour postprandial	2 h PP BS	Chemistry	Blood
Glucose, random	BS	Chemistry	Blood
Glucose tolerance test	GTT	Chemistry	Blood or urine
γ-Glutamyl transpeptidase	GGT	Chemistry	Blood
Glycosylated hemoglobin	HbA_{1c}, GHB, GHB	Chemistry	Blood
Gram stain (smear)		Bacteriology	Any body fluid
Growth hormone	GH or HGH	Chemistry	Blood
Guaiac		Urinalysis/ Feces/ POCT	Urine or stool
Guthrie test (serum phenylalanine)	PKU	Chemistry	Blood
Hanging drop prep (*Trichomonas*)		Bacteriology	Vaginal smear
Haptoglobins		Chemistry	Blood
Heavy metals		Chemistry	Urine
Helicobacter pylori	CLO test	Serology/ POCT	Biopsy specimen
Hematocrit	Hct, Crit	Hematology/ POCT	Blood
Hemoglobin	Hgb	Hematology/ POCT	Blood

Procedure	Abbreviation	Laboratory Division	Specimen
Hemoglobin & hematocrit	H&H	Hematology/ POCT	Blood
Hemoglobin electrophoresis		Chemistry	Blood
Hemogram		Hematology	Blood
Hemosiderin		Chemistry	Urine
Hepatitis A antibody	anti-HAV	Serology	Blood
Hepatitis B core antibody	anti-HB$_c$Ag	Serology	Blood
Hepatitis B surface antigen	HB$_S$Ag	Serology	Blood
Hepatitis B surface antibody	anti-HB$_S$Ag	Serology	Blood
Hepatitis screen (acute)		Serology	Blood
Herpes serology		Serology/ Microbiology	Blood
Herpes simplex virus	HSV	Serology/ Microbiology	Blood/any specimen
Herpes smear		Microbiology	Smear of specified area
Heterophil antibodies screen		Serology	Blood
High-density lipoproteins	HDLs	Chemistry	Blood
Histoplasma, culture		Bacteriology	Sputum
Histoplasma, serology		Serology	Blood
HLA B27 typing		Blood bank	Blood
Homovanillic acid	HVA	Chemistry	Urine
Human chorionic gonadotropin	hCG	Chemistry/ POCT	Blood
Human immunodeficiency virus screen	HIVB$_{24}$AG	Serology	Blood
Human placental lactogen	HPL	Chemistry	Urine
Hydroxybutyrate dehydrogenase	HBD	Chemistry	Blood
17-Hydroxycortico-steroids		Chemistry	Urine
5-Hydroxyindoleacetic acid	5-HIAA	Chemistry	Blood or urine
17-Hydroxysteroids (see 17-Hydroxycortico-steroids)			

Procedure	Abbreviation	Laboratory Division	Specimen
Icterus index		Chemistry	Blood
Immunodiffusion		Chemistry	Blood
Immunoelectro-phoresis	IEP	Chemistry	Blood
Immunoglobulin A	IgA	Serology	Blood
Immunoglobulin E	IgE	Serology	Blood
Immunoglobulin G	IgG	Serology	Blood
Immunoglobulin M	IgM	Serology	Blood
Immunologic pregnancy test	hCG	Urinalysis	Urine (morning specimen)
India ink test		Bacteriology	Cerebrospinal fluid
Indices, red blood cells	RBC Indices	Hematology	Blood
Indirect Coombs'		Blood bank	Blood
Insulin tolerance test		Chemistry	Blood
International Normalized Ratio (used with prothrombin time)	INR (PT-INR)	Hematology	Blood
Iodine uptake	^{131}I	Chemistry	Blood
Iontophoresis (sweat electrolytes)		Chemistry	Sweat
Iron	Fe	Chemistry	Blood
Iron-binding capacity	IBC	Chemistry	Blood
Isocitrate dehydrogenase	ICD	Chemistry	Blood
Isoenzymes (Isozymes)	CK-MB	Chemistry	Blood
Isoenzymes (Isozymes)	CPK or CK	Chemistry	Blood
Ivy bleeding time	Bl time	Hematology	Blood
17-Ketogenic steroids	17 KGS	Chemistry	Blood or urine
Ketones (acetone)		Urinalysis or chemistry	Urine or blood
K&L chains (Bence Jones proteins)		Chemistry	Urine
Lactate (lactic acid)		Chemistry	Blood
Lactate dehydrogenase	LDH	Chemistry	Blood or cerebro-spinal fluid
Lactate dehydrogenase isoenzymes	LDH Iso	Chemistry	Blood
Lactose tolerance test		Chemistry or GI lab	Blood
Lead		Chemistry	Blood or urine

Procedure	Abbreviation	Laboratory Division	Specimen
LE cell prep (see Lupus erythematosus)			
Lee-White coagulation time	Coag time or Lee-White	Hematology	Blood
Legionella culture (Legionnaires' disease)		Microbiology	Bronchial washing
Legionella serology		Serology/ Microbiology	Blood
Leptospira culture		Bacteriology	Urine
Leucine aminopeptidase (also called cytosol aminopeptidase)	LAP	Chemistry	Blood or urine
Leukocyte alkaline phosphatase		Hematology	Blood
Leukocyte count (see White blood cell count)			
Librium level (chlordiazepoxide)		Chemistry	Blood
Lipase		Chemistry	Blood
Lipid phenotype		Chemistry	Blood
Lipoprotein electrophoresis		Chemistry	Blood
Lithium level	Li	Chemistry	Blood
Low-density lipoproteins	LDLs	Chemistry	Blood
Lupus erythematosus	LE cell prep	Hematology	Blood
Luteinizing hormone	LH	Chemistry	Blood
Luteinizing hormone– releasing factor	LHRF	Chemistry	Blood
Macroglobulin		Chemistry	Blood
Magnesium	Mg or Mg⁺	Chemistry	Blood
Melanin		Urinalysis or chemistry	Urine
Mercury	Hg	Chemistry	Urine
Metanephrine		Chemistry	Urine
Methemoglobin		Chemistry	Blood
Microglobulin β_2 (see β_2-Microglobulin)			
Mixed lymphocyte culture		Serology	Blood
Monospot (see Heterophil antibodies screen)			

Procedure	Abbreviation	Laboratory Division	Specimen
Myoglobin		Chemistry	Urine
Nasopharyngeal culture	N-P culture	Bacteriology	Nose swab
Neutral fat (lipid profile fractionation)		Chemistry or GI lab	Blood
5'-Nucleotidase		Chemistry	Blood
Occult blood		Urinalysis/ Micro- biology/ POCT	Urine or stool
17-OH corticosteroids (see 17-Hydroxycortico- steroids)			
Orinase tolerance test		Chemistry	Blood
Osmolality		Chemistry	Blood or urine
Osmotic fragility, RBCs		Hematology	Blood
Ova and parasites	O&P	Parasitology	Stool
Packed-cell volume (see Hematocrit)			
Pancreatic cytology		Cytology	Pancreatic fluid
Pap smears and stains		Cytology	Many body areas, such as cervix and stomach
Parasites, schistosomes		Parasitology	Stool or urine
Parathyroid A&B		Chemistry	Blood
Parathyroid hormone	PTH	Chemistry	Blood
Partial thromboplastin time	PTT	Hematology	Blood
Peak & Trough Level (many drugs)		Toxicology	Blood
Peritoneal fluid smear		Cytology	Peritoneal fluid
pH		Chemistry/ POCT	Blood, urine, or stool
Phenobarbital level		Chemistry	Blood
Phenolsulfonphthalein	PSP	Chemistry	Urine
Phenothiazine level		Chemistry	Blood or urine
Phenylalanine (see Guthrie test)			
Phospholipids		Chemistry or GI lab	Blood
Phosphorus	PO_4	Chemistry	Blood or urine

Procedure	Abbreviation	Laboratory Division	Specimen
Phosphatase, acid (see Acid phosphatase)			
Phosphatase, alkaline (see Alkaline phosphatase)			
Pinworm		Parasitology	Scotch tape prep
Pituitary gonadotropin	FSH	Chemistry	Blood
Placental lactogen, human	HPL	Chemistry	Urine
Plasma cortisol		Chemistry	Blood
Plasma osmolality		Chemistry	Blood
Platelet adhesion study		Hematology	Blood
Platelet aggregation		Hematology	Blood
Platelet concentrate		Blood bank	Blood
Platelet count	Plts or Plt ct	Hematology	Blood
Polymerase chain reaction	PCR	Serology	
Porphobilinogen		Chemistry	Urine
Porphyrins		Chemistry	Urine
Porter-Silber chromogens (see 17-Hydroxycortico-steroids)			
Potassium	K	Chemistry	Blood or urine
Pregnanediol		Chemistry	Urine
Pregnanetriol		Chemistry	Urine
Progesterone		Chemistry	Blood or urine
Prolactin		Chemistry	Blood
Pronestyl level (procainamide)		Chemistry	Blood
Prostate-specific antigen	PSA	Chemistry	Blood
Prostatic acid phosphatase	PAP	Chemistry	Blood
Protein (cerebrospinal fluid)		Chemistry	Cerebrospinal fluid
Protein (urine)		Urinalysis	Urine
Protein-bound iodine	PBI	Chemistry	Blood
Protein electrophoresis		Chemistry	Blood
Protein, total		Chemistry	Blood
Proteus Ox-19		Serology	Blood
Prothrombin time	PT, pro-time	Hematology	Blood
Quantitative urine culture (colony count)		Bacteriology	Urine

Procedure	Abbreviation	Laboratory Division	Specimen
Quinidine level		Chemistry	Urine
Rapid plasma reagin	RPR	Serology	Blood
Red blood cells	RBCs	Hematology	Blood
Red cell distribution width	RDW	Hematology	Blood
Red cell fragility		Hematology	Blood
Red cell indices	RBC indices	Hematology	Blood
Red cell morphology	RBC morph	Hematology	Blood
Red cell survival		Chemistry	Blood
Renin		Chemistry	Blood
Respiratory syncytial virus	RSV	Virology	Blood or nasopharyngeal or sputum
Reticulocyte count	Retics	Hematology	Blood
RH factor		Blood bank	Blood
RH globulin workup		Blood bank	Blood
Rheumatoid factor	RA	Serology	Blood
Rubella antibody		Serology	Blood
Rubella, culture		Bacteriology	Blood
Rubeola, culture		Bacteriology	Blood
Salicylate level		Chemistry	Blood or urine
Schilling's test		Chemistry	Urine
Secretin		Chemistry	Duodenal secretions
Secretin with pancreatic cytology		Cytology or GI lab	Duodenal secretions
Sedrate (see Erythrocyte sedimentation rate)			
Semen		Urinalysis	Semen
Serotonin, serum		Chemistry	Blood
Serotonin, urine	5-HIAA	Chemistry	Urine
Serum glutamic-oxaloacetic transaminase	SGOT (see AST)	Chemistry	Blood or cerebro-spinal fluid
Serum glutamic-pyruvic transaminase	SGPT (see ALT)	Chemistry	Blood
Serum protein electrophoresis	SPE	Chemistry	Blood
Sickle cell prep		Hematology	Blood
Sodium	Na	Chemistry	Blood, urine, or sweat
Sputum, culture		Bacteriology	Sputum

Procedure	Abbreviation	Laboratory Division	Specimen
Staphylococcus aureus	TCT (tube coagulase test)	Bacteriology	Blood, pharyngeal, etc.
Stool, culture		Bacteriology	Stool
Stool for ova and parasites	O&P	Microbiology	Stool
Strychnine		Chemistry	Urine
Sulfa level		Chemistry	Blood
Sweat chloride		Chemistry	Sweat
Sweat electrolytes (Na and Cl)		Chemistry	Sweat
Tegretol level (carbamazepine)		Toxicology	Blood or urine
Template bleeding time	TBT	Hematology	Blood
Testosterone		Chemistry	Blood
Theophylline level		Toxicology	Blood
Thrombin clotting time	TCT	Hematology	Blood
Thromboplastin time, activated partial (see Activated partial thromboplastin time)			
Thyroid antibody titer	TAT	Serology	Blood
Thyroid-binding globulin	TBG	Chemistry	Blood
Thyroid globulin antibody		Serology	Blood
Thyroid-stimulating hormone	TSH	Chemistry	Blood
Thyroxine	T_4	Chemistry	Blood
Tobramycin level		Toxicology	Blood
Total iron binding capacity	TIBC	Chemistry	Blood
Total lipids		Chemistry or GI lab	Blood
Total protein	TP	Chemistry	Blood, urine, or cerebrospinal fluid
Toxicology screen		Toxicology	Blood, urine, or gastric contents
Toxoplasma		Serology	Blood
Triglycerides		Chemistry	Blood
Triiodothyronine resin uptake	T_3	Chemistry	Blood

Procedure	Abbreviation	Laboratory Division	Specimen
Troponin		Chemistry	Blood
Tuberculosis culture	TB AFB	Bacteriology	Sputum, urine, or cerebro-spinal fluid
Type & X-match		Blood bank	Blood
Type & screen	T&S	Blood bank	Blood
Typhoid o&h		Bacteriology	Blood
Urea clearance		Chemistry	Blood or urine
Urea nitrogen	BUN	Chemistry	Blood or urine
Uric acid		Chemistry	Blood or urine
Urinalysis	UA	Urinalysis	Urine
Urine culture	UC	Microbiology	Urine
Urine reflex		Urinalysis/ Microbiology	Urine
Urobilinogen		Urinalysis/ Chemistry	Urine or stool
Uroporphyrins		Chemistry	Urine
Vaginal smear		Cytology	Vaginal smear
Vanillylmandelic acid	VMA	Chemistry	Urine
Venereal Disease Research Laboratories	VDRL (see RPR)	Serology	Blood
Vitamin B_{12} (see Schilling's test)			
Washed cells		Blood bank	Blood
White blood cell count	WBC	Hematology	Blood
Whole blood		Blood bank	Blood
Wound culture		Bacteriology	Any wound

The National Association of Health Unit Coordinators (NAHUC) Standards of Practice and Code of Ethics

Standards of Practice for Health Unit Coordinators

Standard 1—Education
Health unit coordinator personnel shall be prepared through appropriate education and training programs for their responsibility in the provision of non-direct patient care and non-clinical services.

Standard 2—Policy and Procedure
Written standards of health unit coordinators' practice and related policies and procedures shall define and describe the scope and conduct of non-clinical service provided by the health unit coordinator. These standards, policies, and procedures shall be reviewed annually and revised as necessary. These revisions will be dated to indicate the last review, signed by the responsible authority, and implemented.

Standard 3—Standards of Performance
Written evaluation of health unit coordinators shall be criteria based and related to the standards of performance as defined by the health care organization.

Standard 4—Communication
The health unit coordinator shall appropriately and effectively communicate with nursing and medical staff, all ancillary departments, visitors, guests, and patients.

Standard 5—Professionalism and Ethics

The health unit coordinator shall take all possible measures to assure the optimal quality of non-direct, non-clinical patient care. The optimal professional and ethical conduct and practices of NAHUC members shall be maintained at all times.

Standard 6—Leadership

The health unit coordinator shall be organized to meet and maintain established standards of non-clinical services.

Code of Ethics for Health Unit Coordinators*

Members shall conduct themselves in such a manner as to gain the respect and confidence of the patients, health care personnel, and community, as well as respecting the human dignity of each individual.

Members shall protect the patient's rights, including the right to privacy.

Members shall strive to achieve and maintain a high level of competency.

Members shall strive to improve their knowledge and skills by participating in educational and professional activities and sharing the benefits of their attainments with their colleagues.

Unethical and illegal professional activities shall be reported to the appropriate authorities.

---

*From National Association of Health Unit Coordinators, Code of Ethics, 2007, with permission.

APPENDIX **G**

Notes

Notes

Notes

Notes

Glossary

Following is a list of terms that are discussed throughout Chapters 1 through 22 in *LaFleur Brooks' Health Unit Coordinating*, 6th edition. The number of the chapter in which the term is introduced appears after each definition.

Accepting Assignment   Providers of medical services agreeing that the receipt of payment from Medicare for a professional service will constitute full payment for that service (2)

Accountability   Taking responsibility for your actions, being answerable to someone for something you have done (6)

Accreditation   Recognition that a health care organization has met an official standard (2)

Ace Wraps   Elastic gauze used for temporary compression to various parts of the body to decrease swelling and skin breakdown (11)

Active Exercise   Exercise performed by the patient without assistance as instructed by the physical therapist (17)

Activities of Daily Living   Tasks that enable individuals to meet basic needs (e.g., eating, bathing) (17)

Acuity   Level of care a patient would require based on his or her medical condition, used to evaluate staffing needs (3)

Acute Care   Short-term care for serious illness or trauma (2)

Admission Day Surgery   Surgery for which the patient enters the hospital on the day of surgery; it may be called *same-day surgery* or *A.M. admission* (19)

Admission Service Agreement or Conditions of Admission Agreement   Form signed upon the patient's admission that sets forth the general services that the hospital will provide; also may be called *conditions of admission, contract for services,* or *treatment consent* (19)

Admixture   The result of adding a medication to a container of intravenous solution (13)

Advance Directives   Documents that indicate a patient's wishes in the event that the patient becomes incapacitated (19)

Adverse Drug Event   Injury or harmful reaction that results from the use of a drug (13)

Aerobic   Living only in the presence of oxygen (17)

Aerosol   Liquid suspension of particles in a gas stream for inhalation purposes (17)

Afebrile   Without fever (10)

Ageism   Discrimination on grounds of age (5)

Aggressive Behavioral style in which a person attempts to be the dominant force in an interaction (5)

Airborne Precautions/Isolation Required use of mask and ventilated room, in conjunction with standard precautions (22)

Allergy Acquired, abnormal immune response to a substance that does not normally cause a reaction; may involve medications, food, tape, and many other substances (8)

Amniocentesis Needle puncture into the uterine cavity performed to remove amniotic fluid, the liquid that surrounds the unborn baby (14)

Ampoule (Ampule) Small glass vial sealed to keep contents sterile; used for subcutaneous, intramuscular, and intravenous medications (13)

Anorexia Nervosa Intense fear of gaining weight or becoming fat, although underweight (12)

Antibody Immunoglobulin (protein) produced by the body that reacts with and neutralizes an antigen (usually a foreign substance) (14)

Antigen Any substance that induces an immune response (14)

Apical Rate Heart rate obtained from the apex of the heart (10)

Apnea Cessation of breathing (16)

Apothecary System Ancient system of weight and volume measurements used to measure drugs and solutions (13)

Aquathermia Pad Waterproof plastic or rubber pad connected to a bedside control used to apply heat or cold (also called a *K-Pad* or a *water flow pad*) (11)

Arterial Blood Gases (ABGs) Diagnostic study to measure arterial blood gases (oxygen and carbon dioxide) to gather information needed to assess and manage a patient's respiratory status (16)

Arterial Line (art line) Catheter placed in an artery that continuously measures the patient's blood pressure (11)

Assertive Behavioral style in which a person stands up for his or her own rights and feelings without violating the rights and feelings of others (5)

Attending Physician Term applied to a physician who admits and is responsible for a hospital patient (2)

Auscultation The act of listening for sounds within the body to evaluate the condition of the heart, blood vessels, lungs, pleura, intestines, or other organs, or to detect the fetal heart sound (17)

Autologous Blood The patient's own blood donated previously for transfusion as needed by the patient; also called *autotransfusion* (11)

Automatic Stop Date Date on which specific categories of medications must be discontinued unless renewed by the physician (13)

Autonomy Independence; personal liberty (6)

Autopsy Examination of a body after death; may be performed to determine the cause of death or for medical research (20)

Axillary Temperature Temperature reading obtained by placing the thermometer in the patient's axilla (armpit) (10)

Bariatrics Field of medicine that focuses on the treatment and control of obesity and diseases associated with obesity (19)

Bariatric Surgery Surgery performed on part of the gastrointestinal (GI) tract as treatment for obesity (19)

Bedside Commode Chair or wheelchair with an open seat, used at the bedside by the patient for the passage of urine and stool (10)

Biopsy   Tissue removed from a living body for examination (14)

Blood Gases   Diagnostic study to determine the exchange of gases in the blood (16)

Blood Pressure   Measure of the pressure of blood against the walls of the blood vessels (10)

Body Mass Index (BMI)   Body weight in kilograms divided by height in square meters. This is the usual measurement used to define overweight and obesity (12)

Bolus   Concentrated dose of medication or fluid, frequently given intravenously (13)

Brainstorming   Structured group activity that allows three to ten people to tap into the creativity of the group to identify new ideas. Typically in quality improvement, the technique is used to identify probable causes and possible solutions for quality problems (7)

Broken Record   Assertive skill, wherein a person repeats his or her position over and over again (5)

B-scan   Image made up of a series of dots, each indicating a single ultrasonic echo. The position of a dot corresponds to the time elapsed, and the brightness of a dot corresponds to the strength of the echo (16)

Bulimia Nervosa   Recurrent episodes of binge eating (rapid consumption of a large amount of food in a discrete period of time) and self-induced vomiting, with use of laxatives or diuretics (12)

Caloric Study   Test performed to evaluate the function of cranial nerve VIII. It also can indicate disease in the temporal portion of the cerebrum (16)

Calorie   Measurement of energy generated in the body by the heat produced after food is eaten (11)

Capillary Blood Gases (CBG)   Diagnostic study performed primarily on infants. Blood is obtained from the infant's capillary arterial vessel, usually from the heel (16)

Capitation   Payment method whereby the provider of care receives a set dollar amount per patient regardless of services rendered (2)

Capsule   Gelatinous single-dose container in which a drug is enclosed to prevent the patient from tasting the drug (13)

Cardiac Arrest   The patient's heart contractions are absent or insufficient to produce a pulse or blood pressure; also may be referred to as *code arrest* (22)

Cardiac Monitor   Monitor of heart function that provides a visual and audible record of heartbeat (16)

Cardiac Monitor Technician   One who monitors patient heart rhythms and notifies the registered nurse (RN) of rhythm changes (additional training required); often done in conjunction with health unit coordinator responsibilities on a telemetry unit (1, 16)

Cardiac Pacemaker   Electronic device, temporary or permanent, that regulates the pace of the heart when the heart is incapable of doing so (17)

Cardiac Stress Test   Noninvasive study that provides information about the patient's cardiac function (16)

Cardiopulmonary Resuscitation (CPR)   Basic life-saving procedure of artificial ventilation and chest compressions done in the event of a cardiac arrest (all health care workers are required to be certified in CPR) (7)

Career Ladder Pathway of upward mobility (1)

C-Arm Mobile fluoroscopy unit used in surgery or at the bedside (15)

Case Manager Health care professional and expert in managed care who assists patients in assessing health and social service systems to ensure that all required services are obtained; also coordinates care with doctor and insurance companies (2)

Catastrophic Coverage Coverage that a Medicare beneficiary has after reaching a certain quantity of "out of pocket" monies paid for their medications during the temporary coverage gap. The beneficiary will pay a coinsurance amount (such as 5% of the drug cost) or a copayment ($2.15 or $5.35 for each prescription) for the rest of the calendar year (2)

Cathartic Agent that causes evacuation of the bowel (laxative) (15)

Catheterization Insertion of a catheter into a body cavity or organ to inject or remove fluid (11)

Celsius Scale used to measure temperature in which the freezing point of water is 0° and the boiling point is 100° (formerly called *Centigrade*) (21)

Census List of all occupied and unoccupied hospital beds (7, 19)

Centers for Disease Control Division of the U.S. Public Health Service that investigates and controls diseases that have epidemic potential (22)

Central Line Catheter or Central Venous Catheter (CVC) Large catheter that provides access to the veins and/or to the heart to measure pressures; catheter is threaded through to the superior vena cava or right atrium; used for administration of intravenous therapy (13)

Central Service Department Charge Slip Form that is initiated to charge a discharged patient for any items that were not charged to him at the time of use (7)

Central Service Department Credit Slip Form that is used to credit a patient for items found in the room unused after the patient's discharge, or if it is found that a patient was mistakenly charged for an item that was not used for that patient (7)

Central Service Department Discrepancy Report List of items that are missing from the nursing unit patient supply cupboard or closet that were not charged to a patient; it is sent to the nursing unit from the central service department each day (8)

Certification The process of testifying to or endorsing that a person has met certain standards (1)

Chiropractic Medicine A complementary and alternative health care profession with the purpose of diagnosing and treating mechanical disorders of the spine and musculoskeletal system with the intention of affecting the nervous system and improving health (2)

Chronic Care Care for long-duration illnesses such as diabetes or emphysema (2)

Clean Catch (CC) Method of obtaining a urine specimen through a special cleansing technique; also called a *midstream urine* (14)

Clinical Death Occurs when no brain function is present (20)

Clinical Decision Support System (CDSS) Computerized program that provides suggestions or default values for drug doses, routes, and frequencies. The program also may perform drug allergy checks, drug–laboratory value checks, drug interaction checks, and so forth (1, 2)

Clinical Indications (CI)   Notations recorded when diagnostic imaging is ordered, to indicate the reason for doing the procedure (15)

Clinical Pathway   Method of outlining a patient's path of treatment for a specific diagnosis, procedure, or symptom (3)

Clinical Tasks   Tasks performed at the bedside or in direct contact with the patient (1)

Code Blue   Term used in hospitals to announce when a patient stops breathing or when their heart stops beating, or both (7)

Code of Ethics   Set of standards for behavior based on values (6)

Code or Crash Cart   Cart stocked by the nursing and pharmacy staff with emergency medication, advanced breathing supplies, intravenous solutions and appropriate tubing, needles, a heart monitor and defibrillator, an oxygen tank, and a suction machine (used when a patient stops breathing, when their heart stops beating, or both) (7)

Color Doppler   Enhanced form of Doppler echocardiography in which different colors are used to designate the direction of blood flow (16)

Communicable Disease   Disease that may be transmitted from one person to another (22)

Community Health   Emphasis on prevention and early detection of disease for members of a community (2)

Comorbidity   The presence of one or more disorders (or diseases) in addition to a primary disease or disorder, or the effect of such additional disorders or diseases (19)

Compression Garment   Tight-fitting, custom-made garment used to put constant pressure on healed wounds to keep down scarring (11)

Compressor Grip (C-GRIP)   Tight, stretchy, tubular material used for temporary compression (17)

Computed Tomography (CT)   Radiographic process of creating computerized images (scans) of body organs in horizontal slices (15)

Computer on Wheels (COW)   Computer on a cart with wheels that can be taken into patients' rooms (4)

Computer Physician Order Entry (CPOE)   Computerized program into which physicians directly enter patient orders; replaces handwritten orders on an order sheet or prescription pad (1, 2)

Computerized Medication Cart   Storage cart that requires confidential user ID and a password to gain access to medications (13)

Computerized Nurses' Notes   Documentation entered directly into the patient's electronic medical record, usually at the patient's bedside on a portable computer (3)

Confidentiality   Keeping private any confidential information, spoken or written (6)

Conflict   Emotional disturbance—striving for one's own preferred outcome, which, if attained, prevents others from achieving their preferred outcomes (5)

Continuous Quality Improvement (CQI)   The practice of continuously improving quality at each level of each department of every function of the health care organization (also called total quality management [TQM]) (7)

Contrast Media   Substances (solids, liquids, or gases) used in diagnostic imaging procedures that permit the radiologist to distinguish between different body densities; they may be injected, swallowed, or introduced by rectum or vagina (15)

Coroner's Case A death that occurs because of sudden, violent, or unexplained circumstances, or a patient who expires during the first 24 hours after admission to the hospital (20)

Crackle Common, abnormal respiratory sound that consists of discontinuous bubbling noises heard on auscultation of the chest during inspiration (also called *Rale*) (17)

Crisis Stress Profound effect experienced by individuals as the result of common, uncontrollable, often unpredictable life experiences (e.g., death, divorce, illness) (7)

Cultural Differences Factors such as age, gender, race, socioeconomic status, and so forth (5)

Culturally Sensitive Care Care that involves understanding and being sensitive to a patient's cultural background (5)

Culture A set of values, beliefs, and traditions that are held by a specific social group (5)

Culture and Sensitivity The growth of microorganisms in a special medium (culture), followed by a test to determine the antibiotic to which they best respond (sensitivity) (14)

Custodial Care Care and services of a nonmedical nature, which consist of feeding, bathing, watching, and protecting the patient (20)

Cytology The study of cells (14)

Daily Laboratory Tests Tests that are ordered once by the doctor but are carried out every day until the doctor discontinues the order (14)

Damages Monetary compensation awarded by a court for an injury caused by the act of another (6)

Dangle The patient sits and dangles their feet over the edge of the bed (10)

Decoding Process of translating symbols received from the sender to determine the message (5)

Defendant Person against whom a civil or criminal action is brought (6)

Defibrillation Application of an electrical shock to the myocardium through the chest wall to restore normal cardiac rhythm (17)

Deposition Pretrial statement of a witness under oath, taken in question-and-answer form as it would be in court, with an opportunity given to the adversary to be present to cross-examine (6)

Diagnosis-Related Group (DRG) Classification system used to determine payments from Medicare based on assignment of a standard flat rate to major diagnostic categories. This flat rate is paid to hospitals regardless of the full cost of the services provided (2)

Dialysis Removal from the blood of wastes usually excreted by the kidneys (17)

Dietary Reference Intake (DRI) Framework of nutrient standards now in place in the United States. These provide reference values for use in planning and evaluating diets for healthy people (12)

Dietary Supplement Product (other than tobacco) taken by mouth that contains a "dietary ingredient" intended to supplement the diet. Dietary supplements come in many forms, including extracts, concentrates, tablets, capsules, gel caps, liquids, and powders (12)

Differential   Identification of the types of white cells found in the blood (14)

Dipstick Urine   Visual examination of urine with the use of a special chemically treated stick (14)

Direct Admission   A patient who was not scheduled to be admitted and is admitted from the doctor's office, clinic, or emergency room (19)

Disaster Procedure   Planned procedure that is carried out by hospital personnel when a large number of persons have been injured (22)

Discharge Planning   Centralized, coordinated, multidisciplinary process that ensures that the patient has a plan for continuing care after leaving the hospital (20)

Discrimination   Seeing a difference; prejudicial treatment of a person (6)

Document Management System (DMS)   Computer system (or set of computer programs) used to track and store electronic documents and/ or images of paper documents (4)

Document Scanner   Device used to transmit images of paper documents/pictures to be entered into the patient's electronic record (4)

Donor-Specific or Donor-Directed Blood   Blood donated by relatives or friends of the patient to be used for transfusion as needed (11)

Doppler Ultrasound   Procedure used to monitor moving substances or structures, such as flowing blood or a beating heart. Used to locate vessel obstructions, to observe fetal heart sounds, to localize the placenta (afterbirth), and to image heart functions (16)

Downtime Requisition   Requisition (paper order form) used to process information when the computer is not available for use (4)

Dumbwaiter   Mechanical device used to transport food or supplies from one hospital floor to another (4)

Dysphagia   Difficulty eating/swallowing (12)

Dyspnea   Difficult or labored breathing (17)

Echocardiogram (2D M-mode Echo)   Diagnostic, noninvasive procedure in which ultrasound is used to study the structure and motion of the heart (16)

Egg-Crate Mattress   Foam-rubber mattress (11)

Elective Surgery   Surgery that is not emergency or mandatory and can be planned at a time of convenience (19)

Electrocardiogram (EKG or ECG)   Graphic recording produced by electrical impulses of the heart (16)

Electroencephalogram (EEG)   Graphic recording of the electrical impulses of the brain (16)

Electrolytes   Group of tests done in chemistry, which usually includes sodium, potassium, chloride, and carbon dioxide (14)

Electromyogram (EMG)   Record of muscle contraction produced by electrical stimulation (16)

Electronic Medical Record (EMR)   Electronic record of patient health information generated by one or more encounters in any care delivery setting (1, 2)

Electronystagmography   Test used to evaluate nystagmus (involuntary rapid eye movement) and the muscles that control eye movement (16)

Electrophysiologic Study (EPS) Invasive measure of electrical activity (16)

Elevated Toilet Seat Elevated seat that fits over a toilet with handrails for patients who have a problem sitting on a lower seat (11)

Elitism Discrimination based on social/economic class (5)

Emergency Admission Admission necessitated by accident or a medical emergency; such an admission is processed through the emergency department (19)

Emesis Vomit (10)

Empathy Capacity for participating in and understanding the feelings or ideas of another (6)

Encoding Translating mental images, feelings, and ideas into symbols to communicate them to the receiver (5)

Endoscopy Visualization of a body cavity or hollow organ by means of an endoscope. Gastrointestinal (GI) studies also are performed in the Endoscopy department (16)

Endotracheal Tube (ET Tube) Tube inserted through the mouth that supplies air to the lungs and assists breathing. The ET tube is connected to a ventilator (17)

Enema The introduction of fluid and/or medication into the rectum and sigmoid colon (11)

Enteral Feeding Set Includes equipment needed to infuse tube feeding; includes plastic bag for feeding solution and may be ordered with or without a pump (12)

Enteral Nutrition The provision of liquid formulas into the gastrointestinal (GI) tract by tube or orally (12)

Epidemiology Study of the occurrence, distribution, and causes of health and disease in humans; the specialist is called an *epidemiologist* (22)

Ergonomics Branch of ecology concerned with human factors in the design and operation of machines and the physical environment (7)

Erythrocyte Red blood cell (14)

Esteem Needs A person's need for self-respect and for the respect of others (5)

Ethics Behavior that is based on values (beliefs); how we make judgments with regard to right and wrong (6)

Ethnocentrism Inability to accept other cultures, or an assumption of cultural superiority (5)

Evidence All the means by which any alleged matter of fact, the truth of which is submitted to investigation at trial, is established or disproved; evidence includes the testimony of witnesses and the introduction of records, documents, exhibits, objects, or any other substantiating matter offered for the purpose of inducing belief in the party's contention by the judge or jury (6)

Evoked Potential Studies Tests used to evaluate specific areas of the cortex that receive incoming stimuli from the sensory nerves of the eyes, ears, and lower or upper extremities (16)

Expert Witness Witness who has special knowledge of the subject about which he or she is to testify; the knowledge generally must be such that it is not normally possessed by the average person (6)

Expiration A death (20)

Extended Care Facility Medical facility that cares for patients who require expert nursing care or custodial care (20)

Extravasation Leakage of fluid into tissue surrounding a vein (13)

Extubation Removal of a previously inserted tube (such as an endotracheal tube) (17)

Face Sheet Form initiated by the admitting department and included in the inpatient medical record that contains personal and demographic information; usually computer generated at the time of admission (also may be called the *information sheet* or *front sheet*) (19)

Fahrenheit Scale used to measure temperature in which 32° is the freezing point of water and 212° is the boiling point (21)

Fasting No solid foods by mouth and no fluids that contain nourishment (e.g., sugar, milk) (14)

Febrile Elevated body temperature (fever) (10)

Feedback Response to a message (5)

Feeding Tube Small, flexible plastic tube that usually is placed in the patient's nose and that goes down to the stomach or small intestine to provide and/or increase nutritional intake (12)

Fidelity Doing what one promises (6)

Fluoroscopy Observation of deep body structures that are made visible by the use of a viewing screen instead of film; contrast medium is required for this procedure (15)

Fogging Assertive Skill Skill in which a person responds to a criticism by making noncommittal statements that cannot be argued against (5)

Foley Catheter Type of indwelling retention catheter (11)

Food Allergy Negative physical reaction to a particular food involving the immune system (people with food allergies must avoid the offending foods) (12)

Food and Drug Administration (FDA) U.S. Government agency whose purpose is to ensure that foods, drugs, cosmetics, and medical devices are safe and labeled properly (13)

Food Intolerance A more common problem than food allergies involving digestion (people with food intolerances can eat some of the offending food without suffering symptoms) (12)

Fowler's Position Semi-sitting position (10)

Gastric Suction Used to remove gastric contents (11)

Gastritis Inflammation of the stomach (12)

Gastroenteritis Inflammation of the stomach and intestines (12)

Gastrointestinal Study Diagnostic study related to the gastrointestinal system (16)

Gastrostomy Feeding Feeding by means of a tube inserted into the stomach through an artificial opening in the abdominal wall (12)

Gavage Feeding by means of a tube inserted into the stomach, duodenum, or jejunum, through the nose or an opening in the abdominal wall; also called *tube feeding* (12)

GI Study Diagnostic study related to the gastrointestinal system (16)

Guaiac Method of testing stool and urine using guaiac as a reagent for hidden (occult) blood (also may be called a *Hemoccult slide test*) (14)

Harris Flush or Return Flow Enema Mild colonic irrigation that helps expel flatus (11)

Health Maintenance Organization   Organization that has management responsibility for providing comprehensive health care services on a prepayment basis to voluntarily enrolled persons within a designated population (2)

Health Records Number   Number assigned to the patient on or before admission; it is used for record identification and is used for all subsequent admissions to that hospital (also may be called *medical records number*) (19)

Hemovac   Disposable suction device (evacuator unit) that is connected to a drain inserted into or close to a surgical wound (11)

Heparin Lock Intravenous (IV)   Catheter with a small chamber that is covered with a rubber diaphragm or a specially designed cap and is used to administer medications or to gain venous access in case of an emergency; also called a *Saline Lock* (11, 13)

Hepatitis B Virus (HBV)   Infectious blood-borne disease that is a major occupational hazard for health care workers (22)

Holistic Nursing Care   Modern nursing practice that expresses the philosophy of total patient care and considers the physical, emotional, social, economic, and spiritual needs of the patient; also called *Comprehensive Care* (3)

Holter Monitor   Portable device that records the heart's electrical activity and produces a continuous electrocardiographic (ECG) tracing over a specified period (16)

Home Health   Equipment and services made available to patients in the home to provide comfort and care (2)

Homeopathic Medicine   Alternative medical system. Belief that "like cures like," meaning that small, highly diluted quantities of medicinal substances are given to cure symptoms, when the same substances given at higher or more concentrated doses would actually cause those symptoms (2)

Hospice   Supportive care for terminally ill patients and their families (2)

Hospitalist   Full-time, acute care specialist who focuses exclusively on hospitalized patients (2)

Hostile Environment   Sexually oriented atmosphere or pattern of behavior that is determined to be sexual harassment (6)

HUC Preceptor   Experienced, working health unit coordinator (HUC) selected to train/teach an HUC student or new employee (5)

Human Immunodeficiency Virus (HIV)   Virus that causes acquired immunodeficiency syndrome (AIDS) (22)

Hydration   Adequate water in the intracellular and extracellular compartments of the body (12)

Hydrotherapy   Treatment with water (17)

Hyperbaric Oxygen Therapy (HBOT)   Treatment that involves breathing 100% oxygen while in an enclosed system pressurized to greater than one atmosphere (sea level) (17)

Hypertonic   Concentrated salt solution (>0.9%) (17)

Hypnotics   Drugs that reduce pain or induce sleep; may include sedatives, analgesics, and anesthetics (13)

Hypotonic   Dilute salt solution (0.9%) (17)

Impedance Cardiography (ICG) Flexible and fast-acting noninvasive monitoring system that measures total impedance (resistance to the flow of electricity in the heart) (16)

Implied Contract Nonexplicit agreement that affects some aspect of the employment relationship (6)

Incident Episode that normally does not occur within the regular hospital routine (22)

Incontinence Inability of the body to control the elimination of urine and/or feces (11)

Induced Sputum Specimen Sputum specimen obtained by performing respiratory treatment to loosen lung secretions (17)

Indwelling (Retention) Catheter Catheter that remains in the bladder for a longer period until a patient is able to void completely and voluntarily, or as long as hourly accurate measurements are needed (11)

Infiltration The tip of the intravenous (IV) catheter comes out of the vein or pokes through the vein, and the IV solution is released into surrounding tissue. This also could occur if the wall of the vein becomes permeable and leaks fluid (11)

Informed Consent Doctrine that states that before a patient is asked to consent to a risky or invasive diagnostic or treatment procedure, they are entitled to receive certain information: (1) a description of the procedure, (2) any alternatives to it and their risks, (3) the risks of death or serious bodily disability associated with the procedure, (4) probable results of the procedure, including any anticipated problems with recuperation and time needed for recuperation, and (5) anything else that generally is disclosed to patients who are asked to consent to the procedure (6, 19)

Infusion Pump Device used to regulate flow or rate of intravenous fluid; commonly called an *IV pump* (11)

Ingestion Taking in of food by mouth (12)

Injectables Medications that are given by forcing a liquid into the body by means of a needle and syringe (intra-arterial, intradermal, intramuscular, intravenous, and subcutaneous) (13)

Instillation Slow introduction of fluid into a cavity or passage of the body that should remain for a specific length of time before it is drained or withdrawn; purpose is to expose tissues in the area to the solution, to hot or cold, or to a drug or substance in the solution (13)

Insufflate To blow a gas or powder into a tube, cavity, or organ to allow visual examination, to remove an obstruction, or to apply medication (13)

Intake and Output Measurement of the patient's fluid intake and output (10)

Integrated Delivery Networks Health care organizations merged into systems that can provide all needed health care services under a single corporate umbrella (2)

Interdisciplinary Teamwork Well-coordinated collaboration across health care professionals toward a common goal (i.e., improved, efficient patient care) (3)

Intermittent (Straight) Catheter Single-use catheter that is introduced and kept in place long enough to drain the bladder (5 to 10 minutes) and then is removed (11)

International Statistical Classification of Diseases and Related Health Problems Detailed description of known diseases and injuries. Every disease (or group of related diseases) is described along with its diagnosis and is given a unique code, up to six characters long; published by the World Health Organization (2)

Interpreter Person who facilitates oral communication between or among parties who are conversing in different languages (5)

Intervention Synonymous with treatment (17)

Intramuscular (IM) Injection Injection of a medication into a muscle (13)

Intravenous (IV) Administered directly into a vein (13)

Intravenous Hyperalimentation or Total Parenteral Nutrition (TPN) Method used to administer calories, proteins, vitamins, and other nutrients into the bloodstream of a patient who is unable to eat; must be infused into the superior vena cava through a central line catheter—not given through a peripheral IV catheter (13)

Intravenous Infusion Administration of fluid through a vein (11)

Intubation Insertion and placement of a tube (within the trachea, may be endotracheal or tracheostomy) (17)

Invasive Procedure Diagnostic or therapeutic technique that requires entry of a body cavity or interruption of normal body functions (16)

Irrigation Washing out of a body cavity, organ, or wound (11)

Isolation Placement of a patient apart from other patients insofar as movement and social contact are concerned, for the purpose of preventing the spread of infection (22)

Isometric Of equal dimensions; holding ends of contracting muscle fixed so that contraction produces increased tension at a constant overall length (17)

IV (intravenous) Push (IVP) Method of giving concentrated doses of medication directly into the vein (13)

Jackson-Pratt (JP) Disposable suction device (evacuator unit) that is connected to a drain inserted into or close to a surgical wound (11)

Kangaroo Pump Brand name of a feeding pump used to administer tube feeding (12)

Kosher Adherence to the dietary laws of Judaism; conventional meaning in Hebrew is "acceptable" or "approved" (12)

K-Pad Electric device used for heat application (also called *K-thermia pad, aquathermia pad*, or *aquamatic pad*) (11)

Liability Condition of being responsible for damages resulting from an injurious act or for discharging an obligation or debt (6)

Living Will Declaration made by the patient to the family, medical staff, and all concerned with the patient's care, stating what is to be done in the event of a terminal illness; directs the withholding or withdrawing of life-sustaining procedures (19)

Locator Small tracking device worn by nursing personnel and health unit coordinators so that their location may be detected on the interactive console display when necessary (4)

Love and Belonging Needs A person's need to have affectionate relationships with people and to have a place in a group (5)

Lozenge Medicated tablet or disk that dissolves in the mouth (13)

Lumbar Puncture Procedure performed to remove cerebrospinal fluid from the spinal canal (14)

Magnet Status   Award given by the American Nurses Credentialing Center (ANCC) to hospitals that satisfy a set of criteria designed to measure the strength of their quality of nursing (2)

Magnetic Resonance Imaging   Technique used to produce computer images (scans) of the interior of the body with the use of magnetic fields (15)

Managed Care   Use of a planned and systematic approach to providing health care, with the goal of offering quality care at the lowest possible cost (2)

Manometric Studies   Procedures performed to evaluate certain areas of the body with the use of a manometric device to measure and record pressures; usually performed in the Endoscopy department (16)

Material Safety Data Sheet (MSDS)   Basic hazard communication tool that provides details on chemical dangers and safety procedures (22)

Medicaid   Federal and state program that provides medical assistance for the indigent (2)

Medical Emergency   Emergency that is life threatening (22)

Medical Malpractice   Professional negligence of a health care professional; failure to meet a professional standard of care, resulting in harm to another, for example, failure to provide "good and accepted medical care" (6)

Medical Savings Accounts (MSAs)   Tax-exempt bank accounts that are *owned by an individual* and managed by a financial institution. The individual must have a qualified health plan. An individual cannot use the tax benefits of an MSA until the qualified health plan is in place. The qualified health insurance policy can be completely independent of the MSA (2)

Medicare   Government insurance enacted in 1965 for individuals over the age of 65 or any person with a disability who has received Social Security for 2 years (some disabilities are covered immediately) (2)

Medicare Supplement   Private insurance plan available to Medicare-eligible persons to cover the costs of medical care not covered by Medicare (2)

Medication Administration Record (MAR)   List of medications that each individual patient is currently taking; used by the nurse to administer the medications (13)

Medication Nurse   Registered nurse or licensed practical nurse who administers medications to patients (13)

Menu   List of options that is projected onto the viewing screen of the computer (4)

Merger   Combining of individual physician practices and small, stand-alone hospitals into larger networks (2)

Message   Images, feelings, and ideas transmitted from one person to another (5)

Metastasis   Process by which tumor cells spread to distant parts of the body (15)

Methicillin-resistant *Staphylococcus aureus* (MRSA)   A variation of the common bacteria, *Staphylococcus aureus* (22)

Metric System   System of weights and measures based on multiples of 10 (13)

Microfilm Film that contains a greatly reduced photographic image of printed or graphic matter (18)

M-Mode Echo Image obtained with M-mode echocardiography that shows the motion (M) of the heart over time. 2D M-mode would be a two-dimensional study (16)

Modality Method of application or employment of any therapeutic agent; limited usually to physical agents and devices (15)

Modem Device that enables a computer to send and receive data over regular phone lines (4)

Morbid Obesity Excess of body fat that threatens necessary body functions such as respiration (12)

Name Alert Method of alerting staff when two or more patients with the same or similarly spelled last names are located on a nursing unit (8)

Narcolepsy Chronic ailment that consists of recurrent attacks of drowsiness and sleep during the daytime (16)

Narcotic Controlled drug that relieves pain or produces sleep (13)

Nasogastric Tube (NG Tube) Tube that is inserted through the nose into the stomach (11)

Naturopathic Medicine Alternative medical system that proposes the existence of a healing power in the body that establishes, maintains, and restores health. Treatments include nutrition and lifestyle counseling, nutritional supplements, medicinal plants, exercise, homeopathy, and treatments from traditional Chinese medicine (2)

Nebulizer Gas-driven device that produces an aerosol (17)

Needleless IV Hep-lock Safe, sharp device that is placed on a peripheral intravenous catheter when used intermittently (11)

Negative Assertion Assertive skill by which a person verbally accepts the fact that they have made an error, without allowing it to reflect on their worth as a human being (5)

Negative Inquiry Assertive skill by which a person requests further clarification of a criticism to get to the real issue (5)

Negligence Failure to satisfactorily perform one's legal duty, such that another person incurs some injury (6)

Nerve Conduction Studies (NCS) Measures how well individual nerves can transmit electrical signals (often performed with an electromyogram) (16)

Neurologic Vital Signs (Neuro-checks) Measurement of the function of the body's neurologic system; includes checking pupils of the eyes, verbal response, and so forth (10)

Nonassertive Behavioral style by which a person allows others to dictate their self-worth (5)

Non-clinical Tasks Tasks performed away from the bedside (1)

Noninvasive Procedure Procedure that does not require entry into the body, as with puncturing of the skin (16)

Nonverbal Communication Communication that is not written or spoken but that creates a message between two or more people through the use of eye contact, body language, and symbolic and facial expression (5)

Nosocomial Infection Infection that is acquired from within the health care facility (22)

Nuclear Medicine Technique that uses radioactive materials to determine the functional capacity of an organ (15)

Nursing Intervention   Any act by a nurse that implements the nursing care plan or clinical pathway, or any specific objective of that plan or pathway (3)

Nutrients   Substances derived from food that are used by body cells, for example, carbohydrates, fats, proteins, vitamins, minerals, and water (12)

Obesity   Excess amount of body fat usually defined by body mass index (12)

Observation Patient   Patient who is assigned to a bed on the nursing unit to receive care for a period of less than 24 hours; also may be referred to as a *medical short stay* or *ambulatory patient* (19)

Obstructive Sleep Apnea (OSA)   Cessation of breathing during sleep (16)

Occlusion   Blockage in a canal, vessel, or passage of the body (16)

Occult Blood   Blood that is undetectable to the eye (14)

Occupational Safety and Health Administration (OSHA)   U.S. government regulatory agency concerned with the health and safety of workers (22)

Old Record   Patient's record from previous admissions stored in the Health Records department that may be retrieved for review when a patient is admitted to the emergency room, nursing unit, or outpatient department (older microfilmed records may be requested by the patient's doctor) (8)

"On Call" Medication   Medication prescribed by the doctor to be given prior to the diagnostic imaging procedure; the department notifies the nursing unit of the time the medication is to be administered to the patient (15)

One-Time or Short-Series Order   Doctors' order that is executed according to the qualifying phrase, and then is automatically discontinued (9)

Organ Donation   Donating or giving one's organs and/or tissues after death; one may designate specific organs (i.e., only cornea) or any needed organs (20)

Organ Procurement   Process of removing donated organs; may be referred to as *harvesting* (20)

Orthostatic Hypotension   Temporary lowering of blood pressure (hypotension) usually caused by standing up suddenly; also called *postural hypotension* (10)

Orthostatic Vital Signs   Measurement of blood pressure and pulse rate first in supine (lying), then in sitting, and finally in standing position (11)

Over-the-Counter (OTC) Drugs   The FDA defines OTC drugs as safe and effective for use by the general public without a doctor's prescription (13)

Oxygen Saturation   Noninvasive measurement of gas exchange and red blood cell oxygen-carrying capacity (10, 16)

Pacemaker   Electronic device, temporary or permanent, that regulates the pace of the heart when the heart is incapable of doing so (16)

Pap Smear   Test performed to detect cancerous cells in the female genital tract; the Pap staining method also can be used to study body secretions and excretions and tissue scrapings (14)

Paracentesis   Surgical puncture and drainage of a body cavity (14)

Paraphrase   Repeating messages in your own words to clarify their meaning (5)

Patent or Patency   Term that indicates that no clots are present at the tip of the needle or catheter, and that the needle tip or catheter is not against the vein wall (open) (11)

Parenteral Nutrition   Mode of feeding that does not use the gastrointestinal tract; instead, nutrition is provided through intravenous delivery of nutrient solutions (12)

Parenteral Routes   Nonoral methods used for giving fluids or medications (e.g., injection, intravenous approach) (13)

Passive Exercise   Exercise in which the patient is submissive and the physical therapist moves the patient's limbs (17)

Patency   Term that indicates that no clots are present at the tip of the needle or catheter, and that the needle tip or catheter is not against the vein wall (open) (11)

Pathogenic Microorganisms   Disease-carrying organisms that are too small to be seen with the naked eye (22)

Pathology   Study of body changes caused by disease (14)

Patient Account Number   Number assigned to the patient for access to insurance information; usually, a unique number is assigned each time the patient is admitted to the hospital (19)

Patient Care Conference   Meeting that includes the doctor or doctors caring for the patient, the primary nurses, the case manager or social worker, and other caregivers involved in the patient's care (20)

Patient-Controlled Analgesia (PCA)   Medications administered intravenously by means of a special infusion pump controlled by the patient within order ranges written by the doctor (13)

Pedal Pulse   Pulse rate obtained at the top of the foot (10)

Penrose Drain   Drain that that is inserted into or close to a surgical wound and that may lie under a dressing, extend through a dressing, or be connected to a drainage bag or a suction device (11)

Pen Tabs or Tablet PC   Computers that may be removed from their base, or portable computers that can be taken into patient rooms; a stylus is used to enter information directly into a patient's electronic record, as in a notebook (4)

Percutaneous Endoscopic Gastrostomy (PEG)   Insertion of a tube through the abdominal wall into the stomach under endoscopic guidance (12)

Perennial Stress   Wear and tear of day-to-day living with the feeling that one is a square peg trying to fit in a round hole (7, 8)

Perioperative   Pertaining to the time of surgery (17)

Peripheral Intravenous Catheter   Catheter that begins and ends in the extremities of the body; used for the administration of intravenous therapy (11)

Philosophy   Principles; underlying conduct (6)

Physiologic Needs   A person's physical needs, such as the need for food and water (5)

Piggyback   Method by which drugs usually are administered intravenously in 50 to 100 mL of fluid (13)

Plaintiff   Person who brings a lawsuit against another (6)

Plasma Fluid portion of the blood in which the cells are suspended; contains a clotting factor called *fibrinogen* (14)

Plethysmography (Arterial) Usually performed to rule out occlusive disease of the lower extremities; may identify arteriosclerotic disease in the upper extremity (16)

Plethysmography (Venous) Measures changes in the volume of an extremity; usually performed on a leg to exclude DVT (deep vein thrombosis) (16)

Pneumatic Hose Stockings that promote circulation by sequentially compressing the legs from ankle upward, promoting venous return (also called *sequential compression devices*) (11)

Pneumatic Tube System System in which air pressure transports tubes that carry supplies, requisitions, or *some* lab specimens from one hospital unit or department to another (4)

Policy and Procedure Manual Handbook that includes such information as guidelines for practice, hospital regulations, and job descriptions for hospital personnel (1)

Portable X-ray X-ray taken by a mobile X-ray machine that is moved to the patient's bedside (15)

Positive Pressure Pressure greater than atmospheric pressure (17)

Postmortem After death (a postmortem examination is the same as an autopsy) (20)

Postprandial After eating (14)

Power of Attorney for Health Care The patient appoints a person (called a *proxy* or *agent*) to make health care decisions should the patient be unable to do so (19)

Pre-admit Process of obtaining information and partially preparing admitting forms prior to the patient's arrival at the health care facility (19)

Precept To train or teach (a student or new employee) (5)

Primary Care Nursing One nurse provides total care to assigned patients (3)

Primary Care Physician Sometimes referred to as the *gatekeepers*, these general practitioners are the first physicians to see a patient for an illness (2)

Principles Basic truths; moral code of conduct (6)

Proactive To take action prior to an event to use power, freedom, and ability to choose responses to whatever happens to us, in accordance with personal values (circumstances do not control us, we control them) (7)

Proprietary For profit (2)

Protective Care Another term for *isolation* (22)

Pulse Deficit The difference between the radial pulse and the apical heartbeat (21)

Pulse Oximetry Noninvasive method used to measure the oxygen saturation of arterial blood (10, 16)

Pulse Rate The number of times per minute the heartbeat is felt through the walls of the artery (10)

Quid Pro Quo (Latin) Involves making conditions of employment (hiring, promotion, retention) contingent on the victim, who provides sexual favors (6)

Radial Pulse   Pulse rate obtained at the wrist (10)

Radiopaque Catheter   Catheter coated with a substance that does not allow the passage of X-rays, thus allowing movement of the catheter to be followed on the viewing screen (16)

Random Specimen   Body fluid sample that can be collected at any time (14)

Range of Motion   Range in which a joint can move (17)

Reactive   Taking action or responding after an event happens; circumstances are often in control (7, 8)

Real-Time Imaging   Ultrasound procedure that instantaneously displays a rapid sequence of images (like a movie) while an object is being examined (16)

Receiver   Person who receives the message (5)

Recertification   Process by which certified health unit coordinators exhibit continued personal and professional growth and current competency to practice in the field (1)

Recommended Dietary Allowance (RDA)   Average daily intake of a nutrient that will meet the requirements of nearly all (97% to 98%) healthy people of a given age and gender (12)

Rectal Tube   Plastic or rubber tube designed for insertion into the rectum; when written as a doctors' order, *rectal tube* means insertion of a rectal tube into the rectum to remove gas and relieve distention (11)

Reduction   Correction of a deformity in a bone fracture or dislocation (17)

Reference Range   Range of normal values for a laboratory test result (14)

Registration   Process of entering personal information into the hospital information system to enroll a person as a hospital patient and create a patient record; patients may be registered as inpatients, outpatients, or observation patients (19)

Rehydration   Restoration of normal water balance in a patient through fluids given orally or intravenously (12)

Release of Remains   Signed consent that authorizes a specific funeral home or agency to remove the deceased from a health care facility (20)

Resident   Graduate of a medical school who is gaining experience in a hospital (2)

Resistive Exercise   Exercise that uses opposition. A T-band or water provides resistance for patient exercises (17)

Respect   Holding a person in esteem or honor; having appreciation and regard for another (6)

Respiration Rate   Number of times a patient breathes per minute (10)

Respiratory Arrest   When the patient ceases to breathe or when respirations are so depressed that the blood cannot receive sufficient oxygen and therefore body cells die (also may be referred to as *code arrest*) (22)

Respondeat Superior (Latin)   "Let the master answer." Legal doctrine that imposes liability upon the employer. *Note:* The employee is also liable for their own actions (6)

Restraints   Devices used to control patients who exhibit dangerous behavior, or to protect the patient (11)

Retaliation   Revenge; payback (6)
Reverse Isolation   Precautionary measure taken to prevent a patient with low resistance to disease from becoming infected (22)
Rhythm Strip   Cardiac study that demonstrates on the electrocardiogram the waveform produced by electrical impulses (16)
Risk Management   Department in the hospital that addresses the prevention and containment of liability regarding patient care incidents (22)
Robotic Surgery   Use of robots in performing surgery (2)
Routine Preparation   Standard preparation suggested by the radiologist to prepare the patient for a diagnostic imaging study (15)
Scan   Image produced with the use of a moving detector or a sweeping beam (scans are produced by computed tomography, magnetic resonance imaging, and ultrasonography) (15)
Scheduled Admission   Patient admission that is planned in advance; may be urgent or elective (19)
Scope of Practice   Legal description of what a specific health professional may and may not do (6)
Self-actualization Need   Need to maximize one's potential (5)
Self-esteem   Confidence and respect for oneself (5)
Serology   Study of blood serum or other body fluids for immune bodies, which are the body's means of defense when disease occurs (14)
Serum   Plasma from which fibrinogen, a clotting factor, has been removed (14)
Sexual Harassment   Unwanted, unwelcome behavior; sexual in nature (6)
Sheepskin   Pad made of lamb's wool or synthetic material; used to prevent pressure sores (used primarily in long-term care) (11)
Sitz Bath   Application of warm water to the pelvic area (11)
Skin Tests   Tests performed to determine the reaction of the body to a substance by observing the results of injecting the substance intradermally or applying the substance topically to the skin. Skin tests are used to detect allergens, to determine immunity, and to diagnose disease (13)
Spirometry   Study undertaken to measure the body's lung capacity and function (16)
Splint   Orthopedic device used for immobilization, restraint, or support of any part of the body that may be rigid (metal, plaster, or wood) or flexible (felt or leather) (17)
Splinting   Holding the incision area to provide support, promote a feeling of security, and reduce pain during postsurgery coughing. A folded blanket or pillow is helpful to use as a splint (11)
Split or Thinned Chart   Portions of the patient's current chart that are removed when the chart becomes so full that it becomes unmanageable (8)
Sputum   Mucous secretion from the lungs, bronchi, or trachea (14)
Standard of Care   Legal duty one owes to another according to the circumstances of a particular case; the care that a reasonable and prudent person would have exercised in the given situation (6)
Standard Precautions   Creation of a barrier between the health care worker and the patient's blood and body fluids (also may be called *universal precautions*) (22)

Standing Order   Doctors' order that remains in effect and is executed as ordered until the doctor discontinues or changes it (9)

Standing PRN Order   Same as a standing order, except that it is executed according to the patient's needs (9)

Stat Order   Doctors' order that is to be executed immediately, then automatically discontinued (9)

Statute   Law passed by the legislature and signed by the governor at the state level and the president at the federal level (6)

Statute of Limitations   Time within which a plaintiff must bring a civil suit; the limit varies depending on the type of suit and is set by the various state legislatures (6)

Stent   Tiny metal or plastic tube that is placed into an artery, blood vessel, or other duct to hold the structure open (17)

Stereotyping   Assumption that all members of a culture or ethnic group act alike (generalizations that may be inaccurate) (5)

Sternal Puncture   Procedure performed to remove bone marrow from the breastbone cavity for diagnostic purposes; also called a *bone marrow biopsy* (14)

Stress   Physical, chemical, or emotional factor that causes bodily or mental tension and may be a factor in disease causation (7)

Subculture   Subgroups within a culture; people with a distinct identity but who have certain ethnic, occupational, or physical characteristics found in a larger culture (5)

Subcutaneous (SQ) Injection   Injection of a small amount of a medication under the skin into fatty or connective tissue (13)

Suppository   Medicated substance mixed in a solid base that melts when placed in a body opening; suppositories are used commonly in the rectum, vagina, or urethra (13)

Surgery Schedule   List of all the surgeries to be performed on a particular day; the schedule may be printed from the computer or sent to the nursing unit by the Admitting department (19)

Suspension   Fine-particle drug suspended in liquid (13)

Swan-Ganz Catheter   Catheter that is placed in the neck or the chest that measures pressures in the patient's heart and pulmonary artery (11)

SWAT HUC, Nurse, or SWAT Team   Health unit coordinator, nurse, or group of health care workers who are on call for all units in the hospital to provide assistance as needed (also may be called *Resource HUC, Nurse,* or *Resource Team*) (3)

Symbols   Notations written in black or red ink on the doctors' order sheet to indicate completion of a step of the transcription procedure (9)

Tablet   Solid dosage of a drug in disk form (13)

Tact   Use of discretion regarding the feelings of others (6)

Tank Room   Room in which hydrotherapy is performed (17)

Ted Hose   Brand name for antiembolism (A-E) hose (11)

Telemetry   Transmission of data electronically to a distant location (16)

Terminal Illness   Illness that ends in death (20)

Therapeutic Diet   Regular diet with modifications or restrictions (also called a *special diet*) (12)

Thoracentesis   Needle puncture into the pleural space in the chest cavity to remove pleural fluid for diagnostic or therapeutic reasons (14)

Timed Specimen   Specimen that must be collected at a specific time (14)

Tissue Typing   Identification of tissue types to predict acceptance or rejection of tissue and organ transplants (14)

Titer   Quantity of substance needed to react with a given amount of another substance; used to detect and quantify antibody levels (14)

Titrate   To adjust the amount of treatment given, to maintain a specific physiologic response (17)

Topical   Direct application of medication to the skin, eye, ear, or other parts of the body (13)

Tort   Wrong against another person or their property that is not a crime but for which the law provides a remedy (6)

Total Parenteral Nutrition (TPN)   Provision of all necessary nutrients via veins (8)

Traction   Mechanical pull on part of the body to maintain alignment and facilitate healing; traction may be static (continuous) or intermittent (17)

Transesophageal Echocardiography (TEE)   Procedure used to assess the heart's function and structures. A probe with a transducer on the end is inserted down the throat (16)

Trendelenburg Position   Position in which the head is low and the body and legs are on an inclined plane (sometimes used in pelvic surgery to displace the abdominal organs upward or out of the pelvis, or to increase blood flow to the brain in hypotension and shock) (10)

Triage   Nursing interventions; classification defined as establishing priorities of patient care, usually according to a three-level model: emergent, urgent, and nonurgent (2)

Tube Feeding   Administration of liquids into the stomach, duodenum, or jejunum through a tube (12)

Tuberculosis (TB)   Disease caused by *Mycobacterium tuberculosis*, an airborne pathogen (22)

Tympanic Membrane Temperature   Temperature reading obtained by placing an aural (ear) thermometer into the patient's ear (10)

Type and Crossmatch   Patient's blood is typed, then tested for compatibility with blood from a donor of the same blood type and Rh factor (14)

Type and Screen   Patient's blood type and Rh factor are determined, and a general antibody screen is performed (14)

Ultrasonography   Technique that uses high-frequency sound waves to create an image (scan) of body organs (also may be referred to as *sonography* or *echography*) (15)

Unit Dose   Any premixed or prespecified dose; often administered with small volume nebulizer (SVN) or intermittent positive-pressure breathing (IPPB) treatments (17)

Urinalysis   Physical, chemical, and microscopic examination of urine (14)

Urinary Catheter   Tube used to remove urine or inject fluids into the bladder (11)

Urine Reflex   Urine is tested; if certain parameters are met, a culture will be performed (14)

Urine Residual   Amount of urine left in the bladder after voiding (11)

Value Clarification   Examination of our value system (6)

Values   Personal belief about worth of principle, standard, or quality; what one holds as most important (6)

Venipuncture Needle puncture of a vein (11)

Ventilator Machine used to give the patient breaths through the endotracheal or tracheostomy tube (17)

Vital Signs Measurements of body functions, including temperature, pulse, respiration, and blood pressure (10)

Void To empty, especially the urinary bladder (11)

Voluntary Not for profit (2)

WALKaroo Another type of computer on a cart on wheels that may be taken into patients' rooms (4)

WALLaroo Chart rack located on the wall outside of a patient's room that stores the patient's chart and when unlocked forms a shelf to write upon (8)

Work Ethics Moral values regarding work (6)

Workable Compromise Working out a conflict in such a way that the solution is satisfactory to all parties (5)

Index

A

Abbreviations
  in activity orders, 61-62
  for all doctors' orders, 157-169
  in diet orders, 70-75
  "do not use" list of, 80-81
  for medications. *See under*
    Medication orders.
  in nursing observation orders, 62
  in nursing treatment orders, 63-70
  in positioning orders, 62
  for surgery, 137-138, 199
ABGs. *See* Arterial blood gases (ABGs).
Accountability, 37
Acquired immunodeficiency
    syndrome (AIDS), 50-51
Activity orders
  abbreviations in, 61-62
  postoperative, 141
Acute hepatitis panel, 102b
Admission procedures
  components in, 132-133, 137
  steps in, 134-136
  for surgical patients, 133-137
Advance directive forms, 42-43
Aerosol treatments, 119-120
Against medical advice (AMA),
    142, 148-149
Aggressive behavioral style, 15, 16t
AIDS. *See* Acquired immunodeficiency
    syndrome (AIDS).
Airborne precautions/isolation, 49-50
Allergy bracelets, 136
AMA. *See* Against medical advice (AMA).
Anesthesia/anesthesiologists' orders, 137
Angioplasty, 115
Antiasthmatic drugs, 119
Antigens, 96-97
Antimicrobial drugs, 119
Aorta, 117f
AP (anteroposterior) position, 104b

*Note: Page numbers followed by f
indicate figures; t, tables; b, boxes.*

Apothecary system, 76-77
Appearance in workplace, 38-39
Arterial blood gases (ABGs), 113
Arterial grafts, 116
Assertive behavioral style, 16t
Assertiveness skills, 15-17
Attitude, 38
Autonomy, 40
Autopsies, 150-151

B

Bacteria
  common nosocomial-related, 48-49
  tests for, 95
  See also specific bacteria.
Bacteriology studies, 88f, 94-95
Basic metabolic panel (BMP), 101b
Beds, patient
  specialty types of, 69
  for traction, 121-122
Behavior. *See* Workplace behavior.
Beneficence, 40
Bias, cultural, 14
Blood
  components of, 67-68, 209-224
  diseases transmitted through, 50-51
  four major blood groups, 98
Blood bank laboratory studies, 88f, 97-98
Blood chemistry studies, 88f, 90-93
Blood glucose monitoring, 70
Blood transfusions
  consent forms for, 139
  diseases transmitted through, 50
  overview of, 67-68
BMP. *See* Basic metabolic panel (BMP).
Body fluids
  disease transmitted through, 50-51
  See also specific body fluids.
Brainstorming, 21
Brand names (drugs), 200-207
"Broken record" communication
    skill, 15
Bronchodilator drugs, 119
Bulletin boards, 29-30

251

CPSIA information can be obtained
at www.ICGtesting.com
Printed in the USA
FSHW021612210420
69338FS